FEEL GREAT, LOSE WEIGHT

Stop Dieting and Start Living

Restore your health through cleansing, proper nutrition, lifestyle changes and emotional healing.

Andreas Moritz

Other books and products
by Andreas Moritz

The Amazing Liver and Gallbladder Flush

Timeless Secrets of Health and Rejuvenation

Cancer Is Not a Disease

Vaccine-nation: Poisoning the Population, One Shot at a Time

Lifting the Veil of Duality

It's Time to Come Alive

Simple Steps to Total Health

Heart Disease No More!

Diabetes—No More!

Ending the AIDS Myth

Heal Yourself with Sunlight

Hear the Whispers, Live Your Dream

Sacred Santémony

Ener-Chi Ionized Stones

Ener-Chi Art

All of the above are available at www.ener-chi.com, www.amazon.com, and
other online or physical bookstores.

FEEL GREAT,
LOSE WEIGHT

Andreas Moritz

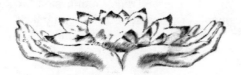

Your Health is in Your Hands

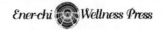

Ener-chi Wellness Press

For Reasons of Legality

The author of this book, Andreas Moritz, does not advocate the use of any particular form of health care but believes that the facts, figures, and knowledge presented herein should be available to every person concerned with improving his or her state of health. Although the author has attempted to give a profound understanding of the topics discussed and to ensure accuracy and completeness of any information that originates from any other source than his own, he and the publisher assume no responsibility for errors, inaccuracies, omissions, or any inconsistency herein. Any slights of people or organizations are unintentional. This book is not intended to replace the advice and treatment of a physician who specializes in the treatment of diseases. Any use of the information set forth herein is entirely at the reader's discretion. The author and publisher are not responsible for any adverse effects or consequences resulting from the use of any of the preparations or procedures described in this book. The statements made herein are for educational and theoretical purposes only and are mainly based upon Andreas Moritz's own opinion and theories. You should always consult with a health care practitioner before taking any dietary, nutritional, herbal or homeopathic supplement, or beginning or stopping any therapy. The author is not intending to provide any medical advice, nor offer a substitute thereof, and makes no warranty, expressed or implied, with respect to any product, device or therapy, whatsoever. Except as otherwise noted, no statement in this book has been reviewed or approved by the United States Food & Drug Administration or the Federal Trade Commission. Readers should use their own judgment or consult a holistic medical expert or their personal physicians for specific applications to their individual problems.

ISBN: 978-0-9821801-7-4

Published by Ener-Chi Wellness Press - Ener-chi.com, U.S.A. (April 2010)
Cover Design/Artwork (Ener-chi Art, Oil on Canvas) by Andreas Moritz

Drinking It In Early
'Unconscious' Addiction
Processed Poison

Introduction

If you've done every diet, taken every pill and read every book, you're probably wondering if there's any point giving it one more shot. But you've possibly been seduced by conventional propaganda that places your health and weight in the hands of weight-loss experts, the gymnasium, medical doctors and the pharmaceutical industry. There's a very definite payoff - for them - in getting vulnerable individuals to believe their self-serving promotional spiel.

But what the universal weight-watcher's guide won't tell you is that losing weight - yes, a considerable amount of weight - is about healing. Despite the notion we've grown up with, that we cannot heal without prescriptions, pills and surgery, conventional wisdom says something else.

Losing weight with the aid of medical props places the power to heal in the hands of practitioners, charlatans and sometimes the Internet. Alternatively, when you take responsibility for your own life, you shift the focal point of healing, from the 'outside' to the 'inside'. And anyone who has done this genuinely and completely will tell you that it works.

Weight loss is an attitude. It is a conscious and active choice. Once you make this all-important shift, it means you are ready to take ownership of yourself, your weight and your life. It means you have truly and intimately acknowledged that you - and only you - have the power to heal yourself.

In this book, we shall discuss the natural way to losing weight - no pill popping, no crash or fad diets, no calorie counting or rigorous aerobic exercise. The human body is a wonderful precision machine that is constantly seeking a state of equilibrium or homeostasis.

In fact, its need for balance is so great that, rather than falling apart, it will bend itself out of shape to accommodate abuse in order to survive.

The greatest threat to this state of equilibrium is toxic abuse from disastrous dietary choices, an erratic lifestyle, chronic stress, constant stimulation of the senses and emotional trauma, to name but a few of the many things we subject our bodies to and still expect to stay in good health.

Practices such as these invariably lead to a state of toxicity. In this book, we shall see how adipose tissue is a defense against mental and emotional toxins. We shall also see why some bodies react to toxicity by turning overweight while others react with cancer or hypertension.

We shall also examine, at the biochemical and physiological level, how careless habits and everyday choices punish and abuse our bodies, how they throw our enzymes, hormones, neurotransmitters, digestive processes and immune system out of gear. By doing this, we turn diseased and obese and blame it on a 'genetic predisposition'.

The good news is that there is a supreme logic and wisdom to the human body, one that we inherited over millions of years during the course of evolution. But we need to create the conditions for the body to function as nature intended it to.

An overweight or obese body is a body in distress. But the human body is also amazingly resilient. So despite the abuse it has been subjected to, it is possible to reverse the processes that led to this state and rebalance the body's biochemistry to achieve its normal, optimal weight.

Sometimes it takes the smallest things. Did you know that mindful eating as opposed to gulping down your food is a simple yet powerful aid to relieving stress and hence shedding excess weight? Or that past traumas and other emotional toxins, quite literally stored in your body's cells, can make you fat?

Alas, we have become so divorced from our own minds and bodies that we often fail to see a simple truth: that a mind and body in harmony with itself and with its surroundings is happy, healthy and of normal weight.

There is indeed a small but growing number of people who are realizing the awesome power within themselves, and unlocking this power to return from a condition of morbid obesity to optimal weight.

It is an amazing and personal journey that you can undertake once you discover just why the very things we dismiss so nonchalantly - eating right, getting a good night's sleep, and remaining physically active - are the very tools that will help you flush out toxins, rebalance your enzymes and hormones, and embrace a healthy lifestyle.

Let me put it this way. If conventional medicine was indeed the panacea we are led to believe it is, why are health budgets ballooning all around? Why are two-thirds of Americans either overweight or obese and the number still rising? And why have so many diet pills or obesity 'wonder drugs' been taken off the market by the federal health authorities?

According to the Centers for Disease Control and Prevention, the average American is already 23 pounds overweight. If the trends of the last three decades continue, researchers estimate that 86 percent of American adults will be overweight by 2030, and by 2048, *every adult American* could be at least mildly overweight.

Obesity is not just a life-threatening condition. It is also very, very expensive. According to some surveys, overweight individuals on average spend $1,400 more a year on medicines than individuals who are not overweight.

Obesity is an expensive illness because of the costs of treating diseases closely linked to this condition - diabetes, heart disease and other ailments - which are common among the overweight.

As for the national budget, surveys in 2009 indicate that obesity-related conditions now account for 9.1 percent of all medical spending, up from 6.5 percent a decade ago. During the same period, the obesity rate rose 37 percent.

In terms of overall costs, after heart disease, cancer and diabetes, obesity-related health spending has reached $147 billion, double what it was a decade ago. And diabetes, a disease closely linked to obesity, costs the US tax-payer $190 billion a year. According to Reed Tuckson of the United Health Foundation, by the year 2018, obesity-related medical expenses will top a staggering $344 billion.

But if we listened to natural wisdom, instead of conventional medicine, we wouldn't be giving away billions of dollars to doctors, hospitals and drug companies to turn our bodies into living chemical laboratories.

We would tune in to our innate wisdom and follow nature's meticulous plan for us. We would heal ourselves.

Chapter 1: The 'Perfect' Myth

Social Selection

It never ceases to amaze me how many weight-loss programs promise 'quick-fix' solutions to shedding pounds and 'amazing tips' to losing weight. But perhaps the websites and programs that surprise me most are those that claim you can lose, say, '10 pounds in 11 days' or '25 pounds in 45 days'.

Apart from the obvious fraudsters looking to make a dishonest buck, there are countless dieticians, nutritionists and weight-reduction programs including gyms and aerobics classes that genuinely shoulder the burden of your excess weight - and promise to help you get rid of it.

Candidates who sign up for these programs are promptly herded onto a weighing scale, a tape measure is thrust around their waist and a diet plan is pushed under their nose, even as a stern finger points to a treadmill or exercise cycle in the gym.

Perhaps some of this desperation 'to cut the flab' has something to do with wanting to have the perfect figure - slim, svelte and sexy for women, and muscular and macho for men.

It is called social selection, where 'beautiful' people, both men and women, are rewarded subtly and not-so-subtly for being slim, trim and 'good looking'. Most of us are conditioned to respond favorably to people who sport a figure that meets certain social standards, and to look askance at anyone who doesn't.

We are constantly bombarded by images of slim and well-toned bodies leaping off billboards, on television, on food packaging, and practically everywhere. But who sets these standards? Who determines what is slim? And is there such as a thing as ideal body weight?

What happens to the millions of overweight and clinically obese people? And not conforming to cosmetic standards is the least of their problems. The health risks that result from being overweight or obese are considerable, never mind the mirror that society holds up to us.

It is a well-known fact that obesity multiplies an individual's risk of heart disease, diabetes and cardiovascular disease, among several other medical conditions. And the excess burden placed on the body and its various systems and organs are only some of the complications that arise from carrying around excess so much baggage.

An individual who weighs more than their optimal weight is suffering from internal pollution, congestion of their internal organs, a toxicity crisis and is carrying around years and years of poisonous debris.

I shall elaborate on the toxicity crisis later in this book but suffice to say for now that even the most scientifically charted weight-reduction plans may have omitted scientific certain vital facts that have little to do with weights and measures, laboratory tests on foods, and calorie counts.

Yes, obesity is a very real problem and it has assumed alarming proportions in the United States. In fact, America has been dubbed a 'nation of overweight people'. Also, obesity ranks among the biggest killers in the US, and childhood obesity, heart disease and diabetes have been areas of concern for a long time.

According to some of the country's premier agencies monitoring health and obesity, more than two-thirds of the American population is overweight and one-third is classified as obese.

In absolute figures, that's over 66 percent of the adult population (more than 200 million people) who qualify as overweight, including 34 percent who are obese, according to the US government's National Health and Nutrition Examination Survey (NHANES) for 2005–2006.

The survey also found that there was a significant increase in these figures over the last two decades. Not surprisingly, this dovetails perfectly with lifestyles becoming more and more sedentary, the personal computer taking over so many chores and other activities that once needed legwork (including outdoor entertainment and sports) and the addiction to fast food and processed foods.

Obesity is also a serious health concern for children and adolescents as well. Data from NHANES surveys (1976–1980 and 2003–2006) shows that an estimated 17 percent of children and adolescents aged 2–19 years are overweight.

Age-wise, the prevalence of obesity for children aged 2–5 years has gone up from 5.0 percent to 12.4 percent; for those aged 6–11 years, from 6.5 percent to 17.0 percent; and for those aged 12–19 years, from 5.0 percent to 17.6 percent.

Weight-Loss Myths

No doubt, most overweight individuals have a desire to lose weight. But sometimes, the desperation is fuelled by the media, the cosmetics industry, pharma companies and food manufacturers. Driven by profit and with no scruples really, these multi-billion dollar industries stand to benefit from your sense of insecurity about your figure and weight.

They make you vulnerable and induce low self-esteem by setting so-called standards of health and encouraging a gullible population to believe that they need to keep shedding pounds to stay healthy and 'look good'.

It is a simple yet beguiling logic that leads millions into a trap from which they cannot escape. Just when you reach the point of desperation, these very industries with their wonder products offer a solution to restore your body back to normalcy and health, and let's not forget, ideal body weight!

As far as corporate predators are concerned, there is only one solution to your dilemma - one or more of the hundreds of weight-loss products they sell either over the counter or as prescription drugs. Notions such as these have led millions of people the world over to adopt a blinkered medical view and self-defeating techniques in their effort to lose weight.

It's somewhat like cultivating a collective psyche that works like magic to the financial gain of a handful of people. It works to pack the shelves of your local grocery store with more and more processed food. It works to create a nation of obese people.

If the food industry and pharma companies didn't do this, who would buy the numerous pills, potions and programs they push to restore you back to a slim state of being?

Exercise and diet are the cornerstones of most weight-reduction programs, so most products and pills relate to these two aspects of health, though there are some imaginative techniques that offer 'super-fast yet safe secrets' to losing weight.

One of these recommendations, followed by millions of overweight people, is that you reduce your calorific intake so that you ingest fewer calories than your body burns in the normal course of the day.

The weight-loss industry has in fact created an entire jargon that cleverly confuses the average intelligent human brain. Visit a dietician and terms such as low-sugar, fat-free, low-carb, low-cal, low-fat and high-fiber are almost certain to haunt your every waking hour.

If it is exercise that you have been advised, then you are likely to be hounded by some positively painful terms such as 'burning fat' while 'building' muscle; 'hitting' the gym; 'high-intensity' exercise; and phrases such as 'no pain-no gain', 'getting enough cardio' and 'going the extra mile'.

Eat less, burn more and punish your body - the message is loud and clear.

Crash Diets: Putting an overweight person on a diet plan seems to bring down anxiety levels instantly. I am not quite so sure what that does to the complex nutritional requirements and overall health of the human body.

Nevertheless, crash diets and starvation diets, which shock the body, are a popular option, such as the famous Atkins Diet, the South Beach Diet and the Weight Watchers' Diet.

In fact, when the Atkins Diet swept across America and many other countries in the late 1990s and early 2000s, it was estimated that 1 in every 11 Americans was on this diet and 18 percent of the population was on a low-carb diet in general.

Sales of carbohydrate-loaded foods such as pasta and rice fell dramatically and there was panic in the food industry, especially among some major brands. Alternatively, as is their wont, some food manufacturers cashed in on the 'low-carb craze', as it was called, and began to market products that were low in carbohydrates (Coke released C2 which supposedly contained half the amount of carbohydrates, sugars and calories as compared to standard Coke!).

But like with all fads, the popularity of the Atkins Diet waned though controversies on the effects of a diet as drastic as this and took a while longer to subside.

Exercise: For those who want to crank it up a little and dieting is not enough, the so-called experts have another formula - exercise furiously *and* follow a crash diet. Somewhere down the line, a miracle is supposed to take place. That is, if you have the stomach, determination and energy levels to exhaust and deplete your body, all at the same time!

Supplements: And there's something for the diet-hungry weight-watcher too - nutritional supplements, vitamin pills and energy drinks! Is it purely coincidental that there should be a readymade solution to almost every weight-watcher's woes?

Diet Pills: Also, can it really be all that simple? Take the darling of the weight-loss industry - diet pills. Straight from the African desert comes a diet pill that acts as an appetite suppressant!

Imagine the excitement this generated in the pharma industry. Finally, modern science had discovered an ancient remedy, a magic pill, to treat obesity! It was an extract of a 'cactiform' plant of the Apocynaceae plant family. Called Hoodia, it contains a chemical compound or glycoside which goes by the innocuous-sounding term 'P57'.

The South African Council for Scientific and Industrial Research (CSIR), which first isolated P57, patented it in 1996. The Council then granted a UK-based company, Phytopharm, a license to synthesize P57 for commercial use.

Phytopharm collaborated with Pfizer on the project but it was later discovered that the drug thus produced led to serious side-effects and damaged the liver. The drug has not been approved by the Food and Drugs Administration (FDA) but it is prescribed and sold illegally, especially online.

Metabolic Enhancers: Metabolic enhancers are another favorite prescription for near-instant weight loss, or so it would seem. According to those who advocate these drugs, metabolic enhancers apparently speed up the body's metabolism and therefore have a strong thermogenic effect. This means there is a sudden increase in body heat, which is supposed to cause lipolysis or the breaking down of fat.

Hypnosis: Another really imaginative quick-fix method to losing weight is, believe it or not, hypnosis! Advocates of this method - who charge exorbitant fees, no doubt - lead one to believe under hypnosis that certain foods are harmful while others are good for you. If only it were really that simple!

Smart Foods: Rivaling hypnosis as a weight-reduction technique is another creative promise to a slimmer way of life - healthy fast foods! Repackaging them as 'smart-foods', advocates of these 'meals for the calorie-conscious' would actually have you believe that McDonald's, Burger King and

Wendy's serve meals that could curb the number of calories you ingest while stopping by at their fast-food outlets.

Claiming that the cattle slaughtered to make burgers has been raised on a fat-free ranch, meals that use these meats can keep your calorific intake in check. No guesses as to who is sponsoring and spreading these incredible notions.

Body Mass Index: Another popular misconception of the weight-watching world is that one size fits all. To devise a standard of reference for weight-watchers and overweight individuals, experts came up with the concept of Body Mass Index or BMI. This is a benchmark used by the Department of Health, weight-loss programs, dieticians and nutritional experts to determine who is overweight and who is not.

Body Type: Mass Belief

BMI is calculated as weight in kilograms divided by height in meters squared, rounded to one decimal place, or weight/height^2 or kg/m$^{2.}$

Adults aged over 20 with a BMI of 25.0–29.9 are classified as overweight and those with a BMI of 30 or more are said to be obese.

Another conventional method to understand body size is to classify it into three body types - ectomorph, mesomorph and endomorph, based on body shape and musculature.

According to the classic definition, the ectomorph is naturally lean and thin and not prone to putting on weight as these individuals have a high metabolic rate. They are overactive and not particularly strong.

The mesomorph is naturally athletic and muscular, naturally lean, loses fat easily and has an efficient and fast-burning metabolism.

The endomorph is podgy and has a rounded body shape. There is a tendency to gain weight and to store fat easily due to a sluggish metabolism.

Even though no dietician or weight-loss plan will actually say this, most weight-reduction methods and crash diets are aimed at converting endomorphs into ectomorphs and mesomorphs.

Haven't you noticed the 'before' and 'after' images used on promotional material for these programs? Quite by magic, women go from being overweight to having the perfect hour-glass figure while men go from downright flabby to trim and muscular.

If only all women who desire to lose weight could be converted into ectomorphs and men into mesomorphs! And yes, most weight-loss programs claim they can indeed perform this simply amazing miracle. If they didn't, who would sign up anyway, right?

A Balanced Body

In this book, we shall explore the principles of good health, and relate them specifically to body weight. Remember, the two are inseparable. You cannot achieve your true optimal body weight if you are not healthy.

According to the ancient science of Ayurveda, every human being is a complex experience or interplay of three processes - mind, body and spirit. All these three together are an expression of your life force or dosha or Prana.

Your every waking and resting moment is therefore an expression of your dosha according to your body type and state of physical, mental and spiritual well-being.

As mentioned above, the human body is traditionally classified into three body types - ectomorph, mesomorph and ectomorph. Ayurveda does not define body type according to musculature. Instead, each of the three body types is a combination of the five elements of the universe - air, fire, water, earth, space.

These body types are Vata, Pitta and Kapha (as explained in detail in my book *Timeless Secrets of Health and Rejuvenation*). Each individual's body type is unique to that individual.

We are all born with some of the characteristics of all three types, but in different proportions. It is therefore important to identify your body type to determine what is good for you and what works for your body.

Good health and happiness is a constant quest for equilibrium. This means that your mind, body and spirit must be in harmony with each other. With time, you will be able to tune in to each of these three aspects of being.

Modern lifestyles, especially in the Western world, have taken us so far from our natural state of good health that we accumulate too much baggage inside.

Stress, processed foods, pill-popping and over-stimulating ourselves have placed a burden on all our body, its organs and systems, and they end up clogged, congested polluted and toxic. The result is a body in distress, struggling in vain to find a sense of balance and equilibrium.

When you contrast this with conventional weight-loss procedures, you will notice that what is good for one person isn't always good for everyone. That is why judging health by common yardsticks doesn't work very well.

For instance, a particular food or even medical drug impacts differently on different people. One size does *not* fit all. Diet plans, exercise regimes and weight-loss programs are tailored to broad classifications. They rarely take into account individual differences.

Also, with their focus on losing weight rather than on health and well-being, they tend to ignore the basic principle - that restoring the body, mind and spirit to its natural equilibrium would result in weight loss *and* a state of vitality and happiness.

A Healthy Body, Normal Weight

Only a healthy body can achieve normal weight. Theories of how much each person should weigh (calculated according to gender, height, ethnicity, etc.) ignore each individual's unique constitutional requirements.

Healthy body weight varies according to individual body types. A healthy Vata type will always be thin, and a healthy Kapha type will always be corpulent and muscular.

The bones of Vatas are light and thinly built, whereas Kaphas have very heavy, dense and compact bones. Both body types have very different, if not completely contradictory, requirements regarding, food, exercise and lifestyles. Pitta types, whose bodies generate more heat, have entirely dissimilar energy requirements to the other body types.

Weight loss for the right reasons i.e. to improve your health, is easy. Trying to shed weight without removing the accumulated toxins first goes against the body's principles of survival and is therefore difficult to achieve.

The body merely protects itself against acid death by keeping the toxins in a neutralized state inside fat cells and bodily fluids.

That is why when you embark on a weight-reduction plan that aims to only help you get rid of excess weight, it often does not work. Only some people actually achieve their goal, and many soon put on the weight they had so painfully shed. With weight being the only criterion, it is somewhat like putting yourself into a mould that was not tailored for you.

It is therefore important to know your body type and then discover your own unique optimal weight. Once you cleanse your body of toxins and accumulated weight and live by the natural principles of healthfulness, weight loss is a natural consequence.

Your health will improve automatically once you remove the toxic waste products and keep the eliminative organs and systems open and clean. The focus needs to be on moving toward good health, rather than on fighting ill health.

Once you have learned the lessons of creating health, you can easily turn your body into a finely tuned instrument that helps you fulfill your desires and lead a life filled with happiness, vitality, abundance and wisdom.

Cleansing Your Body

The human body needs to be cleared of toxins before it can restore itself to its natural weight. Cleansing it also ensures that weight loss takes place smoothly and without leading to adverse effects.

The most powerful and thorough of all the cleansing procedures is the Liver and Gallbladder Flush (described in detail in my book *The Amazing Liver and Gallbladder Flush*). Its most important effect is to restore Agni, the digestive fire (the combined digestive power of all gastrointestinal secretions).

When Agni is stronger, food is digested more efficiently, your body produces less waste and consequently, less waste is deposited in the intestines. However, this can take place only if you also clean out your colon through colonic irrigation or similar colon cleansing methods.

A kidney cleanse ensures that toxins released by the body do not get stuck in the kidneys. The main principle here is that weight loss will take place naturally and without harm if the eliminative organs are first cleared of any accumulated waste deposits. All this will effectively restore the body's health and natural weight.

One liver cleanse, however, will not be sufficient to restore Agni on a permanent basis. You need as many such cleanses as it takes to remove all the accumulated gallstones. After each cleanse, there will be an increase in energy, your abdomen will feel tighter, and you will lose several pounds.

Yet within less than a week, some of the old sluggishness may return and previous food cravings may re-emerge. This shows that gallstones from the rear parts of the liver have traveled forward to exiting bile ducts and clogged up these major bile ducts again, thereby reducing Agni once more. A series of flushes is therefore recommended.

By the time your liver is completely clean, your body weight should be ideal and your energy boundless, provided your diet and lifestyle are healthy and balanced too.

When you analyze the results of all the prominent slimming techniques and dietary plans, you come across one consistent finding. Most people who go on a diet give up before completing it. Of those who continue, only a few lose weight and most of those individuals put the weight back on again. Cleansing the body of accumulated toxins, on the other hand, provides a sound basis for safe and permanent weight loss.

Weight Regulation is Natural

Weight loss occurs spontaneously when the body's natural weight regulation mechanisms are restored. Excessive weight is a symptom of disturbed digestion and metabolism. In addition, it is a sign of chronic toxicity in the body.

Trying to remove the symptom (excessive weight) can be very harmful and disappointing if the accumulated toxins are not removed first. Most weight-reduction programs do not address this vital issue.

The body has a natural resistance to losing excessive weight quickly because sudden weight loss could release a flood of trapped toxins into the bloodstream and even have fatal side-effects such as the collapse of liver functions, kidney failure, and heart attack.

The body never behaves in an irrational way. Weight regulation has to begin by removing the root causes behind the metabolic problems responsible for weight gain.

Boston researchers discovered that people whose pancreas secretes high concentrations of insulin have more difficulty losing weight than those who produce smaller amounts of insulin. This, however, has very little to do with genes, as some doctors may tell you.

The reason 200 million Americans are overweight or cannot shed excess weight is not because of genetic flaws. It is well known that overweight people secrete more insulin. However, over-secretion of insulin is an effect of weight gain, and not its cause.

The reason 200 million Americans are overweight is because they have become insulin resistant. When the insulin receptors of the cells block out insulin, blood sugar begins to rise. To deal with the increase in blood sugar, the pancreas makes more insulin to help remove it from the blood.

One way to deal with this dangerous situation is to have the body convert the excessive amounts of sugar into fat. The more fat a person has accumulated, the less likely he or she is to exercise because this requires effort.

Also, exercising rigorously, as most weight-loss plans recommend, addresses the problem of excess lipid formation; they do not address insulin-resistance or the reason why the body has become insulin resistant.

Insulin also inhibits the body's fat-burning hormone - 'hormone-sensitive lipase'. This hormone is responsible for releasing fat into your bloodstream to be used as fuel. Once this hormone is deactivated, the body can no longer burn fat for energy.

Instead, it must use amino acids and complex sugars stored in the muscles as fuel. This in turn will make you weak and excessively hungry and cause cravings. This creates an endless cycle of increased insulin secretion and fat generation.

To escape this vicious cycle, one must keep the body's insulin secretions low. Low levels of insulin allow your body to produce large amounts of hormone-sensitive lipase, thus burning fat as required. This naturally regulates your weight.

Processed, refined and otherwise manufactured foods all increase insulin levels, and thereby diminish the body's energy reserves.

It is all very simple, really, and does not require any major effort. Discovering and removing the root cause of weight gain is the only way to truly address this problem.

The term 'weight loss' invariably triggers a stress reaction in the body because it is generally associated with rigorous dieting and exercising, neither of which is very palatable. Feeling anxious to lose weight is a recipe for disaster and leads to failure and disappointment.

Besides, despite the many 'guarantees' that these programs offer, you somehow know that these rigid plans have none to offer, really. By the time you reach a point where you are ready to try almost anything, your journey would have led you to discover many people who have tried and stumbled as well as those for whom it hasn't worked.

Alas, there are few if any dieticians and nutritionists pushing weight-reduction programs who actually approach the problem in a holistic way.

Moreover, advocating quick-fix remedies and band-aid treatment and then leaving you in the deep end is convenient. If they didn't produce results 'quickly' and dramatically, it wouldn't be very profitable for these weight-loss experts, would it?

We live in a quick-fix world where we want, and even demand, tangible, visible and instant gains in everything we do. Somewhere along our journey to becoming urbanized and 'developed', we also seem to have lost touch with an intimate part of ourselves—the positive life force that is at the center of our very being.

Chapter 2: Manufactured Obesity

Mind, Not Matter

Eating is central to our existence. Food provides our bodies with energy so that we have enough fuel to run through our day without fatigue setting in. And, of course, we'd like it to taste good too.

But the food we eat also has emotional connotations, not to mention the number of diet plans and opinions nutritionists have to offer. Many individuals who have been on and off weight-reduction plans are so chock-full with information about foods, they could fill an encyclopedia with details on carbohydrates, proteins and fats!

But there are powerful emotional connotations to our eating habits that we rarely pay attention to, and that have as much to do with weight loss or weight gain as the actual foods we eat.

Our eating habits often relate to our body image, how we react to it, and our perception of how others relate to it. If you are overweight, try asking yourself this: Every time you reach for the refrigerator or approach a meal on your plate, are you beset by feelings of anxiety, fear, guilt or shame?

Returning to your optimal weight starts with your beliefs about yourself. Being overweight or obese is about imbalances - in both mind and body. Here, I am not referring to foods that are harmful or unhealthy *per se* but to how you perceive yourself and your body image.

If you think ill of yourself or are uncomfortable with your body image, correcting that perception or imbalance is the true starting point of weight loss. And to heal this imbalance, you have to first love what you don't like for it to heal.

How often have you fallen off the dieting wagon because you've thought your body wouldn't respond anyway? How often have you reached for a burger or chili dog while thinking,

"It doesn't matter, my body won't let go of those extra pounds anyway!"

Being overweight is the body's way of dealing with toxicity. It might sound ironic when you read this but obesity is a constant striving by the body to bring itself back to a state of equilibrium.

Every individual has an optimal weight. Losing weight is therefore all about bringing oneself back to this state of balance in the most natural way. It is about embracing one's body image, oneself and believing that one can be whole again.

This eliminates fear and creates a positive environment for healing, and consequently weight loss. Most diet plans and rigorous exercise programs are driven by fear - fear that any departure from them will either result in weight gain or that one will lose the benefits one has thus far gained.

Fear does *not* create the right environment for weight loss. Happy and healthy beliefs do. The body does not take kindly to radical changes, either in eating habits, exercise or sleep patterns.

Weight loss is therefore about not having to fight any more. It is about believing that you can turn imbalance into a state of equilibrium. This can take place only if you first embrace yourself, and if you believe unconditionally that you have an opportunity to balance the rest of your life and become whole, happy and fulfilled.

This chapter is about understanding why it is so easy to form unhealthy eating habits, the burden they place on the body and why it is profitable for a handful of people to keep a nation of people overweight.

It is also about knowing that the overweight body can restore itself to its optimal and normal weight.

Chemical Warfare

Enemy Number One of the overweight or obese individual is processed foods including fast food, ironically billed as saviors of the 21st century. Breakfast cereals, energy bars, TV dinners, hamburgers, chili dogs, pasta, puddings and baked chicken. You pick them off the shelves, peel off the wrapper, eat most of them on the move or put them in the microwave.

They are time-savers, they are delicious and, why, they are even 'nutritionally enriched'. At least, that's what the label says.

If you can get 'all you need for a healthy start to your day' in a bowl of breakfast cereal, you couldn't ask for more, right? Not so fast. Falling prey to smart advertising spiel and convincing product packaging are more than 75 percent of Americans, whose breakfast consists of bright and colorful cereals.

Hiding behind labels such as 'whole grain', 'high-fiber' and 'nutritionally enriched' are a bag of chemicals - present in all processed foods - dumping chemical toxins into your body.

Starting with your liver, kidneys, small intestine, large intestine or colon and connective tissue, these chemicals - artificial coloring agents, preservatives, food flavoring agents, refined sugars, refined grains, trans fatty acids and even fiber from bran - breakfast cereal could be escalating weight gain and taking your body to a toxicity crisis.

This is easily understood when we take a look at how the body deals with any type of toxin that enters the digestive system. The link between processed foods and weight gain is the liver.

This organ is tasked with more than 500 different functions, two of which are detoxification and burning fat. Apart from neutralizing and rendering toxins harmless, the liver passes on some of the toxins to the colon for elimination. It stores the rest to prevent them from entering the bloodstream.

So the more unnatural chemicals you consume in processed foods, fast food and junk food, the greater the need for detoxification. Your liver is now burdened with this role and is left with little time or energy to burn fat or carry out its other responsibilities.

According to some estimates, three quarters of the average individual's liver is used to store toxins that the liver was unable to render harmless.

When the liver can store no more poison, these chemicals begin to back up into the bloodstream, which sets off another series of harmful reactions in other organs and tissues including the brain.

Apart from promoting weight gain, these additives and preservatives then lead to diseases such as cancer, Alzheimer's disease, heart disease, asthma and neurological disorders.

Colored Poison

Take artificial coloring agents and preservatives, for instance. These chemicals are known to increase hyperactive behavior in preschool children. So if your child suffers from 'hyperkinetic disorder' or Attention Deficit Hyperactivity Disorder (ADHD), eliminate all processed and junk foods from his or her diet.

Food manufacturers never call a spade a spade, nor a coloring agent a coloring agent. Food labels are crafted with care and they camouflage some of the most deadly chemicals we are tempted to ingest.

Some of the chemicals on food labels to watch out for are:

- Sunset yellow, a dye used in, among other foods, orange jellies and squashes, apricot jam and packet soups

- Tartrazine, one of the more controversial coloring additives used in the UK, is another yellow dye used in aerated drinks, ice cream, sweets and jams
- Carmoisine, a red dye, is used in jellies, sweets, blancmanges, marzipan and cheesecake mixes
- Ponceau, also red, is used in European tinned fruit, jellies and salami

Have you ever wondered why food manufacturers so successfully use artificial coloring to tempt you to pick up the food they put out on the shelves - canary yellow bell peppers, ruby red apples, bright yellow corn and emerald broccoli? And, of course, those colorful loops and baubles in breakfast cereal?

This is classic chicanery by which they subtly tap into your innate ability to recognize healthy foods by their colors, an ability that dates back to our evolutionary history.

The human brain is pre-programmed to pick foods that contain usable energy, nutrition and those that boost immunity. These properties are usually present in foods - berries, fruit and vegetables - that are vibrant and brightly colored. It is nature's way of saying, "Come, pick me, I am healthy for you."

What the human body didn't bargain for was artificial colors that play on this innate ability and instead pump your body with toxic chemicals and poisons.

While some of these chemical additives like preservatives increase the shelf life of foods, others kill bacteria, improve taste, replace fats and carbohydrates, and enhance the flavor of processed foods.

Here is some disturbing information. Take a close look at the websites of some of America's biggest fast food restaurants and you will realize that some of the ingredients in those sumptuous meals and salads have more in common with products in your local hardware store than your grocery store!

Among these food additives are artificial coloring agent titanium dioxide (also used in sunscreen), and flavor enhancer monosodium glutamate (MSG), which promotes obesity.

Flavor of Fat

MSG is in fact one of the most poisonous chemical additives in processed and fast foods. It is a carcinogenic neurotoxin that also goes by the name 'processed free glutamic acid' on food labels.

Laboratory mice fed MSG become grotesquely obese and were found to have lesions in the hypothalamus of the brain - the part of the brain that regulates appetite, metabolism or energy balance, and therefore weight gain.

Not surprisingly, this flavor enhancer is also one of the most easily concealed additives and appears on food labels under many innocuous-sounding names: hydrolyzed vegetable protein, autolyzed protein, plant protein extract, textured protein, yeast extract, yeast food, malt extract, broth, stock, seasoning, accent and gelatin.

Another favorite hiding place for MSG in dietary supplements, which are processed foods used by vegetarians, is the label 'organic'. Clever, isn't it?

That is why a vegetarian burger is not the healthy vegetarian burger you think it is. Not by a long shot. Remember this the next time you stop by Burger King. According to the fast food chain's website, its Veggie Burger has six ingredients disguising MSG. Going by the labels soy protein isolate, yeast extract, calcium caseinate, hydrolyzed corn, natural flavors and even 'spices'!

What is the biological link between MSG and obesity? This artificial flavor enhancer, present in soups, gravies and salad dressing, is an excitotoxin, which stimulates the nerve cells to the point of exhaustion, cell damage and eventual cell death.

At the cellular level, metabolizing MSG releases formaldehyde (the same chemical used to store organs and fetuses in biology laboratory jars!) as a byproduct. The formaldehyde then binds with cellular DNA and damages it. Over a period of time, damaged DNA leads to various diseases including cancer.

When consumed in high doses, as in persons who consistently eat a lot of processed foods or junk food, MSG crosses the blood brain barrier and enters the brain. The hypothalamus, the portion of the brain linked to energy regulation and obesity, has no blood-brain barrier and MSG has been shown to cause lesions in the hypothalamus of laboratory mice, which also turn grossly obese.

And it is not only the brain's cells that are vulnerable to MSG. Glutamate receptors to which MSG readily binds, are present across the nervous system, heart, and intestinal tract. So the cell damage caused by this excitotoxin that makes your potato chips taste so delicious can extend to tissues all over the body.

Research on baby formula has revealed the presence of MSG, suggesting that the average American's preoccupation with feeding infants formula could set up an entire generation of children with a tendency to being overweight.

According to some experts, the type of obesity linked to excitotoxins is not linked to food intake. This, they suggest, could explain why some obese people find it difficult to lose excess weight by limiting the amount of food they eat or their fat and calorific intake.

America is a nation practically raised on processed foods and fast foods. And with MSG being one of the most prevalent food additives used in them, it doesn't take a genius to guess why America is a nation of obese people.

No Free Lunches!

When we talk of obesity as being among the top health concerns in America, what better place to start than with school children? Apart from what they are being fed at home, don't we also need to take a look at what children are being served for lunch in school?

The National School Lunch Program was launched in 1946 to help farmers sell surplus produce while also providing nutritious meals to school children. Schools are reimbursed by the US Department of Agriculture (USDA) for every lunch they serve - $2.57 for a free lunch, $2.17 for a reduced-price lunch and 24 cents for a paid lunch.

However, somewhere down the line, flavored and colored processed food and even fast food - chicken nuggets, pizza and energy bars - began finding their way to the school lunch tray, foods that critics point out are promoting obesity and diabetes in school children.

While the USDA justifies parceling out cheesy, meaty and greasy foods to children, critics point out that the Federal government has been quick to oblige food companies, whose leftovers are ending up on the unsuspecting youngsters' lunch trays.

It took $9 billion to feed 30 million school children in 2007, a considerable price to pay for promoting obesity, heart disease and a host of other illnesses in kids. Advocacy groups have been lobbying hard against this but have come up against food lobbies who are loathe to forfeiting their own free lunches! This at a cost of millions and billions of dollars that come from taxpayers' money to fund the National School Lunch Program!

The good news is that some advocacy groups have been able to demonstrate that schools can be in charge of their own menus and kitchens. Some schools, for instance, in Berkley, California, and in Hawaii, are using USDA commodities but are cooking food from scratch and adding organic fruits and vegetables from local farms.

Sweet Surrender

They are sold under simple names like Equal, NutraSweet and Splenda. But artificial sweeteners - notoriously low-calorie or zero-calorie - are highly toxic chemicals. Yet they are among the most widespread additives used in at least 6,000 consumer foods and beverages sold worldwide.

Sample just how powerful they are: Saccharin is more than 400 times as sweet as regular sugar, aspartame is 200 times as sweet, and neotame appears to have super strength sweetness and is thus dubbed 'super aspartame'.

Sucralose, branded as Splenda, is another popular sweetener. No wonder they are the darling of 'diet' drinks companies: zero-calorie, yet powerfully sweet.

As you read this section on sweeteners, consider this following sample of foods and beverages that contain this toxic chemical. According to some estimates, you can pick as many as 600 foods and drinks off the grocery store shelves that have been flavored with aspartame.

Some of these are gum and mints; various types of desserts; milk shakes; medical drugs, food and vitamin supplements; instant teas and coffees, breakfast cereals, and diet beverages including colas.

Among the popular sweeteners, aspartame has received the most attention for two reasons. First, the extremely controversial circumstances under which it was approved by the Reagan administration.

The late American President Ronald Reagan was a 'friend' of G D Searle & Co, the firm that then held the patent for aspartame and was earning billions of dollars from marketing it to the cola giants. Remember, this was when the processed foods and beverages industry was growing into the multi-billion dollar industry it is today.

Second, the avalanche of complaints and protests from patients and the medical fraternity about its side-effects.

The effects of aspartame are documented by the US Food and Drugs Administration's (FDA) own data. In 1995, the agency was forced, under the Freedom of Information Act, to release a list of 92 aspartame symptoms reported by thousands of victims. In 1996, the FDA stopped taking complaints and now denies the existence of the report!

Aspartame has three primary ingredients: aspartic acid, phenylanine, and methanol (or wood alcohol). It also produces a toxic byproduct called diketopiperazine. This sweetener acts on the nervous system in much the same way as MSG does.

It is an excitotoxin, which results in massive cell damage and cell death. Just like MSG, aspartame has been linked to lesions in the hypothalamus and therefore to obesity.

Many overweight individuals who crave colas take refuge, so to speak, in 'Diet' colas. That's because Diet colas ostensibly do not contain the high-calorie sweetener high-fructose corn syrup. But the next time you reach for one of those 'smart drinks', remember one little word - aspartame - and the many diseases you could be inviting.

Researchers and doctors have found that aspartame acts as a slow poison as the side-effects could take several years to manifest themselves. Among the most frequent symptoms are vision loss; memory loss; obesity; testicular, mammary and brain tumors; seizures, coma, and cancer.

Worse still, the symptoms of aspartame poisoning appear to mimic the symptoms of certain major diseases such as fibromyalgia, multiple sclerosis, lupus, ADHD, diabetes, Alzheimer's disease, chronic fatigue, and depression. This makes it very difficult to diagnose.

Aspartame is a synergistic methanol poison, and methanol is known to cause serious birth defects and major developmental disorders such as autism and attention deficit in the offspring of aspartame users.

Despite these devastating research and empirical findings, clever advertising campaigns have managed to make the world believe that aspartame and all the other artificial sweeteners are just simple, harmless, food additives that lend foods and beverages a sweet and delicious taste while helping you keep slim, or even shed some extra pounds.

But here is the double-whammy for individuals who are overweight: Not only is Diet soda not a diet product, but a chemically altered, multiple sodium (salt) and aspartame-containing product that actually makes you crave for carbohydrates and gain weight. It contains formaldehyde, which is stored in the fat cells, particularly in the hips and thighs. A bag of potato chips, anyone?

Sweet Lies, Bitter Truth

What makes cola the developed world's most popular drink? Wily marketing (some would say big fat lies), for sure. It's ironic that intoxicating and addictive marketing could contribute to two of America's most worrying epidemics - obesity and diabetes.

If health experts and doctors could label the contents in a bottle of cola, this is how it would read: Pesticides; carcinogenic preservatives (sodium benzoate); toxic flavor enhancers (MSG); toxic artificial sweeteners in 'diet beverages' (aspartame); ladles of sugar in regular beverages (sucrose and high-fructose corn syrup); a neurotoxin (caffeine); unnatural synthetic vitamins in 'healthful' products; and scores of class-action lawsuits.

But why do colas make us put on weight? The answer lies in four innocuous-sounding words: high-fructose corn syrup (HFCS). Present in most soft drinks and processed foods, HFCS is a refined sugar that has one sole purpose: sweetening a product.

While doing so, it adds plenty of empty calories to our bodies (calories that have zero nutrition, unlike natural sugar) and makes you put on weight.

HFCS, the most popular synthetic sweetener and sugar substitute in the US, is made from corn. It is made by using genetically modified enzymes to convert corn starch into glucose, which is then converted into fructose.

It is no secret that HFCS is directly linked to weight gain. Experts also say it is the single-most significant factor contributing to America's obesity 'epidemic'. But how exactly does HFCS make you fat?

This sweetener piles on the calories, which are directly converted into fat. It also raises the triglyceride levels in the bloodstream.

But there is something more diabolical at work. HFCS fails to trigger the satiety response that kicks in when you eat other foods. Instead, it tricks your brain into believing that the body needs to eat more. In contrast, when you eat carbohydrates that are converted into glucose, the pancreas releases insulin to metabolize the glucose. You also feel full and stop eating.

But when you drink a can of cola, the HFCS does not stimulate the pancreas to produce insulin. It also fails to raise the levels leptin, a hormone produced by the body's fat cells.

When leptin is released into the bloodstream, it acts on the hypothalamus (which regulates energy metabolism) to generate the satiety response. This signals the brain that you have ingested sufficient calories and need to stop eating.

HFCS also does not lower levels of ghrelin, a growth hormone that also increases hunger and appetite.

Drinking colas therefore throws your metabolism out of gear and fails to trigger the signals that turn off appetite and control body weight. You therefore tend to crave colas and drink more and more of the deliciously deceptive sweet stuff.

Interestingly, processed food and beverage companies began to replace liquid cane sugar with HCFS in their products in the 1970s, at the same time when America's obesity problem began to balloon. Researchers say this is no coincidence.

Corn is one of America's three main crops (corn, cotton and soya) and promoting HFCS kept the farm lobby happy. Statistics indicate that between 1970 and 2000 (average annual consumption of HFCS was 73.5 pounds per person), obesity figures in the US went from 15 percent to engulfing one-third of the population.

Remember, cola, which contains 8–10 teaspoons of sugar or 130–150 calories, is just one of the many sources of refined sugar we ingest. Total the sugar intake of the average American, including refined sugar, high-fructose corn syrup and artificial sweeteners, and the shocking intake is 142 pounds a year, or roughly 2.5 pounds per week, according to a report by CBS Broadcasting in June 2007. This figure has risen 23 percent in the last 25 years and is a major cause of soaring rates of obesity and diabetes.

The good news is that HFCS is not harmful in itself. This means it does not produce permanent changes in body chemistry, should you halt its intake in time. Hence, should you kick the cola habit, the food cravings it tends to fuel will diminish.

The bad news is that even if you kick the cola habit, HFCS is hard to avoid because it is used in most processed foods. It is cheap, it blends easily with other ingredients, it extends shelf life, it prevents freezer burn, and it keeps bread soft. It is used in ketchup and even low-fat yoghurt!

Over 40,000 different food items now occupy the shelves of modern grocery stores and 98 percent of them have nothing to do with what nature intended us to eat. Our digestive system has no way to make use of foods robbed of their natural, intrinsic life energy or manipulated and processed to the point of uselessness, regardless of the wonderful ingredients listed on their product labels.

If foods are made in a laboratory, as most of them are, you can no longer consider them food. Instead, they have turned into poison. And poisoning our systems starts early in life, when we are children.

Children make up a large proportion of the sugar-consuming population. And childhood obesity figures are equally alarming (*See Chapter 13*: Burden Of Legacy). Obesity among children aged 12 to 19 went up from 4.2 percent in 1970 to 15.3 percent in 2000 (when consumption of HFCS increased).

Add to this the increasingly sedentary lifestyles among children and it paints an even unhealthier picture. Children spend an average five to six hours a day on sedentary activities, including watching television, using the computer, and playing video games.

Today's children are bombarded and brainwashed with well-crafted TV ads from fast-food chains and other purveyors of high-fat, high-sugar meals and snacks.

But being untruthful to lure young cola addicts is a tactic cola companies have been accused of time and again. In July 2009, in Australia, Coca-Cola was forced to clarify its position with regard to misleading claims it had made in an advertising campaign called 'Motherhood & Myth-Busting'.

The ad campaign, contested by the Australian Competition and Consumer Commission, had popular Australian actor Kerry Armstrong promoting Coke as being 'kiddie-safe'.

Coke had claimed that it was debunking the 'myths' that its cola was 'full of added preservatives and artificial colors'; that it 'makes you fat'; that 'it was originally green'; that 'Coca-Cola contained cocaine once upon a time'; that it was 'packed with caffeine'; and that it 'rots your teeth'.

The bitter truth is that colas, by their very definition, contain significant amounts of preservatives, caffeine, and refined sugar, among other ingredients.

A California study, whose results were released in September 2009, concluded that drinking one or more colas a day increases your chances of obesity by 27 percent. The study also found a stunning 62 percent of adults who drink at least one cola each day are either overweight or obese.

Utterly Butterly Healthy

Most diet plans and nutritionists will tell you that butter is a definite no-no for anyone who wants to lose weight. So this will come as a surprise - butter may have slimming benefits.

But before we go into the details, here's something to think about first. Heart disease rose to become the number one killer in the US between the 1920s and 1960s, about the same time that butter consumption fell from an average 18 pounds per person per year, to four.

Though butter would have to be eliminated as the culprit, it was still tainted as the villain contributing to heart disease, obesity and diabetes, three of America's biggest health concerns today.

So was it pure coincidence that margarine manufacturers had stepped in to convince the gullible public that they had found a healthy substitute for butter? Could margarine have been the unlikely culprit?

Butter provides your body with essential fatty acids, it keeps your hormones in balance, it is good for the heart, it sharpens vision, and it keeps skin moist. So when you eliminate butter from your diet, you are also harming your health.

Butter, used in ancient cultures as an offering to the gods, is a natural food - organic, raw butter is the best form of butter. Cultured raw butter, made from fermented cream, is even healthier.

Margarine, on the other hand, is a processed or 'plastic-like' food, made chemically from refined polyunsaturated oils and hydrogenated to make it viscous.

Here are 10 reasons why organic, raw butter constitutes a healthy addition to your diet:

1. It helps the body absorb Vitamin A which is needed for thyroid and adrenal health
2. It contains lecithin, which helps metabolize cholesterol
3. It contains anti-oxidants which guard against free radicals
4. It strengthens the immune system
5. It is a great source of Vitamins E and K
6. It is a rich source of selenium, a vital mineral
7. Its saturated fats guard against tumors and cancer
8. Vitamin D in butter is essential to calcium absorption

9. It is a rich source of iodine
10. It guards against gastrointestinal infections

But what is wrong with factory-made butter? Factory-made butter is made from pasteurized milk or cream and is nutritionally deficient.

Pasteurization is a process that uses heat to kill harmful bacteria and other organisms. However, it also destroys the 'good' bacteria; it destroys active enzymes, reduces vitamin content, and denatures fragile milk proteins.

But where can you get raw butter? The sale of raw butter is prohibited in the US but it is easy to make at home.

It's All in the Oil

Here's something else that will surprise you. Just like raw butter, coconut oil is not only healthy, it also has slimming properties. If you're looking to lose weight, you're looking for organic, unrefined, extra-virgin coconut oil.

Unlike refined oils, virgin coconut oil contains unrefined essential fatty acids (except Omega 3 and 6 fatty acids which you can get from other sources) that have several health and powerful slimming benefits.

Most of the oil we use to cook our food with is refined oil. To increase shelf life, manufacturers remove the fatty acids - and with that, its main nutrients - from the oil. In fact, a lot of the 'healthy' oils in health food stores lack essential fatty acids (EFAs) and are nutritionally deficient.

The average adult can safely consume about 3.5 tablespoons of coconut oil per day in their diet without the risk of putting on weight. But start slow and gradually increase the quantity you consume.

Coconut oil is made up of medium-chain fatty acids, which are easy to digest and therefore speed up metabolism. On the other hand, long-chain fatty acids (in polyunsaturated oils) take longer to break down and are easily stored as fat in the body.

Some studies even indicate that medium-chain fatty acids also burn fat stored in the body.

Here is how coconut oil can help you lose weight. This virgin oil slows digestion and keeps you feeling full for a longer time. This discourages snacking.

Carbohydrates cooked in coconut oil take longer to be broken down and digested and hence blood glucose or blood sugar levels tend to remain stable and not fluctuate, precipitating further hunger.

Virgin coconut oil is rich in lauric acid, a medium-chain EFA. Lauric acid is a good anti-viral, anti-bacterial and anti-yeast agent, and kills all major strains of Candida albicans. Lauric acid also reduces carbohydrate cravings.

Coconut oil is also a wonderful detoxification agent. It cleanses the body of toxins, keeps the digestive tract healthy, and nourishes the cells in your body. All of this is essential on the road to restoring your body's optimal weight.

Detoxifying the body with coconut oil is important to weight loss because it dissolves and removes toxins trapped in fatty deposits, thereby making fat accumulation increasingly unnecessary. Remember, fat accumulates as a survival mechanism to store toxins engulfed within fatty tissue.

This may also explain why coconut oil helps to build lean muscle, and is preferred by body builders, personal trainers and Olympic athletes.

'Good' and 'Bad' Oils

Understanding fats and oils is a complicated subject, or so the food industry would have you believe. Thanks to propaganda by food and oil manufacturers, we are brainwashed into believing that saturated fats are bad and unsaturated fats are good.

This is not true. There are just as many saturated fats that are healthy for your body as there are unhealthy unsaturated fats. The only factor that determines whether a fat is good or bad for your health is whether it is present in its natural form or is engineered or 'refined'.

When margarine and other refined and hydrogenated products were introduced into the US food market, commonly used coconut oil, flax oils and fish oils disappeared from the shelves of America's grocery stores.

The campaign by the emerging food industry against natural oils and beneficial fats such as coconut oil was fuelled by massive media disinformation that blamed saturated fats for the wave of heart attacks that suddenly began to scare the American population.

For 30 or more years, coconut oil and other healthy oils vanished off the shelves of grocery stores before they made a recent comeback in health food stores. They were replaced by cheap junk oils, including soy oil, cottonseed oil and rapeseed oil (sold as Canola oil).

These refined oils are responsible for severe gastrointestinal disturbances including acid reflux disease, irritable bowel syndrome Crohn's disease, constipation, and colon cancer.

Healthy oil is needed to keep the body's trillions of cells healthy and functioning properly. Their plasma membrane, an active player in glucose absorption, needs to contain a complement of *cis type w=3* unsaturated fatty acids.

This makes cell membranes fluid, allowing them to easily absorb glucose molecules for energy generation. This, in turn, balances blood sugar levels.

By regularly eating fats and oils that are heat-treated (in contrast with natural expeller-pressed oils and untreated fats), cell membranes begin to lose their healthy fatty acids and replace them with harmful trans-fatty acids.

As a result, the cell membranes become thicker, stiffer and stickier, and inhibit the glucose transport mechanism, resulting in elevated blood sugar levels. This sets off a chain reaction, affecting several organs and systems.

To deal with the high blood sugar, the pancreas releases extra insulin, which can lead to inflammation throughout the body. The liver tries to convert some of the excess sugar into fat, stored by adipose cells. This can make the body fat.

To get rid of the rest of the sugar in the blood, the urinary system goes into overdrive. Eventually, the body enters a condition of chronic exhaustion due to the lack of cellular energy.

The adrenal glands respond by pumping extra quantities of stress hormones into the blood, creating mood swings, anxiety and depression. The endocrine glands also malfunction.

Overtaxed by the constant demand for extra insulin, the pancreas fails to produce enough. Body weight may increase a little more each day. The heart and lungs become congested and fail to deliver oxygen to all the cells in the body, including the brain.

Practically every organ and system in the body is affected by this simple dietary mistake.

Chapter 3: The Inside Story

Your physical health and well-being are more intimately connected to your gut and bowels than you may think. After all, that's where it all begins and ends - with digestion and elimination and, of course, everything in between.

To put it simply, what we take in, how we process it and what we keep inside rather than eliminate have everything to do with the diseases we suffer from. Obesity is one of the more direct and obvious consequences of being driven towards what I call a 'toxicity crisis'.

Add to this the mind-body connection and it lends a whole new dimension. The very same processes apply to the human mind - the thoughts and feelings that preoccupy us, how we deal with them and the things we find hard to let go of and that build up as emotional toxins (*See Chapter 4:* The Big Three).

In a perfect world, the mind and body would act in tandem to produce health and happiness. But what happens when the intestines and lymphatic system get polluted and congested?

Obesity is usually the result of internal pollution and congestion starting with the liver, small intestine, bowel and finally the lymphatic system (*See Chapter 3:* The Inside Story). Of course, it is a little more complex than that but there is no escaping the fact that individuals who are overweight are actually poisoning themselves.

Conventional weight-loss experts would have you believe that it is the food you eat and amount of exercise you get that determine whether you are overweight or not, and how you can shed the extra pounds. It is called the 'calories-in, calories-out' approach to weight loss.

These 'professionals' suggest that you adopt complex and sophisticated diets and they even have impressive mathematical formulae to count the calories you gain and lose at every stage.

Throw in some common-sense advice about regular eating habits and sleeping well and often you end up with the perfect weight-loss plan. Or so they would have you believe.

While it is a fact that the food you eat is critical in determining whether you stay healthy or not, burning fat or calories through vigorous exercise is absolutely unnecessary. Neither is pushing the limits of physical endurance, which is brutal and suggests that you care very little for your body.

Most of all, conventional weight-reduction programs address only what you see, that is, the symptoms of disease - a fatty roll under the diaphragm, belly fat, 'love handles' and cellulite on the upper arms and thighs. Of course, there is a different set of exercises for every body part that has piled on excess adipose.

What these weight-loss programs fail to address is the cause of obesity. Why does the body feel the need to put on pounds? What is it defending itself against? And what kind of toxicity crisis is it reeling under?

Dynamic Energy

Powering our very existence is the life force or chi or Prana, digesting your food is Agni or the digestive fire, and determining the movement of fluids and energy in your tissues, organs, muscles and bloodstream are the three doshas - Vata, Pitta and Kapha (*See Chapter 12:* Energize, Not Exercise).

Each dosha is distinguished from the other by its type of energy, the biological processes it governs and natural rhythms and cycles.

Disturbances in the natural energy that flows through your body and keeps you alive cause imbalances in digestive functions, waste disposal and immunological processes. This eventually leads to a state of internal pollution and congestion.

When the liver, stomach, intestines, bowels and lymphatic systems accumulate toxins, they get poisoned, they harden, they get distorted, and they lose their natural shape and functions in a futile attempt to adjust to this new but unhealthy internal environment.

This is the beginning of obesity, gastrointestinal problems and a number of other diseases like cancer. Before we explore these processes and the consequences of their malfunctioning on obesity, let me tell you something that might surprise you.

Did you know that gallstones can lead to severe back pain? Not only does a severely congested gallbladder lead to a fatty liver and the accumulation of weight around the midriff, it also causes spasmodic pain attacks in the back region.

Is it purely coincidental that over 60 percent of Americans are estimated to have back problems and about the same percentage of Americans are overweight? Both conditions are characterized by a digestive system that is malfunctioning, choking, backing up and in distress.

As you see, the root causes of many symptoms and diseases, even obesity, are often not obvious. There is a supreme logic and rhythm to every biological process and the interactions between all of them. But addressing them in a symptomatic way as allopathic medicine does, separates you even further from the causes.

As you continue to read, you will realize that the human body is constantly searching for equilibrium. When things are out of gear, the body then tries to compensate by quite literally bending itself out of shape.

This happens till it can no longer take the overload - the toxicity crisis boils over - and manifests itself as disease. To provide you with a clearer and more comprehensive picture of the disease process, I have included some of the basic insights of Ayurvedic Medicine, which is the most ancient and complete system of natural health care.

Once you understand how illness is 'created', you will also understand how to reverse it.

Digestion: Centre of Existence

The digestive process actually begins in your mouth. Here, food is pre-digested by saliva, which also signals to your pancreas and small intestine that a meal is on the way.

These organs then release the appropriate types and amounts of digestive enzymes and minerals needed to break down the food into the smallest nutrient components.

Not only is it necessary to chew every morsel thoroughly so that it is pre-digested properly, but research suggests that chewing also reduces the release of stress hormones.

Eating a meal - which means you're ingesting calories - is usually a stressful event for individuals who are overweight. This in turn leads to anxiety, fear and insecurity, which tends to make one chew even faster.

Once the food enters your stomach, your salivary enzymes continue to digest it in this organ for as much as an hour. Only then does your stomach begin to secrete its gastric juices - hydrochloric acid, enzymes, mineral salts, mucus and water.

The acid kills harmful microbes and parasites that are naturally present in the food as well as harmful substances such as food additives and chemicals. Also, special enzymes are released to act on proteins.

Once saturated with sufficient acid, the food is pumped into the small intestine which is approximately 6 meters or 18 feet long. This coiled tube-like organ is responsible for most of the chemical digestion and absorption of nutrients, salt and water.

Simultaneously, the liver pours in bile and the pancreas contributes digestive enzymes, minerals and water to further break down starches. Bile, on the other hand, metabolizes fats and proteins.

Metabolized nutrients are absorbed through the walls of the small intestine and pass into the blood, which carries them to the liver for detoxification. The rest are detoxified by the lymphatic system.

The body's complex metabolic processes are powered by Agni, or the 'digestive fire' that 'cooks' the food and its nutrients as they are being processed. Agni is fuelled by bile, without which none of the other digestive juices would be sufficiently effective to break down food into its nutrient components.

There is no underestimating the role of bile, which in a congested environment leads to the formation of gallstones that contribute to sickness and weight gain. Bile, which is alkaline, dilutes the hydrochloric acid. This makes it possible for the intestine to secrete the necessary digestive enzymes for metabolism.

An intestinal pH-value of high acidity would block enzyme secretion and become a major stumbling block for the proper digestion of food. As long as bile secretion from the liver's bile ducts and the gallbladder remain unimpeded by gallstones, good digestion is almost guaranteed, provided that you eat food that is fresh and wholesome.

Refined carbohydrates, refined sugars and chemical additives in processed foods and beverages significantly lower Agni. None of these substances were intended by nature to be ingested and anything that is unnatural, and worse still, consumed regularly and in vast quantities, blocks the digestive fire.

This is where the toxicity crisis, and roots of obesity, begins. When Agni is low, undigested food cannot pass through the intestinal walls into the bloodstream. It becomes a target for destructive bacteria and starts fermenting and putrefying in the intestine.

A chain reaction is set off involving destructive bacteria, toxins and poisonous gases that further impair digestive functions. Over time, the intestine's ability to absorb nutrients is greatly diminished.

More and more toxins and waste is generated, and this increasingly congests the gastrointestinal tract, not to mention the damage it also causes to the liver on rebound. At this stage, food turns into poison.

Here is an astonishing fact: one-third of the Western world's population has been diagnosed with intestinal problems. Take a look at the average American's diet and lifestyle, and that should tell you why.

The mind-body connection is clearly demonstrated by the small intestine. The cerebral cortex of the brain, which controls thought, is intimately connected with the digestive process. Hence, not only foods, but also thoughts need to be properly 'digested' or processed so that they don't cause us any harm.

Undigested thoughts have a poisonous effect on the body as a whole and on the digestive system in particular. Fear, anger, shock, trauma, anxiety and other negative emotions may be locked up in the cellular memory of the intestines for a long time and without any obvious indication of their presence.

Once they have reached a certain degree of concentration, they may suddenly erupt and alter one's personality in a negative way. This can be damaging to the body as well.

In other words, if you feel frequently upset, angry, worried or simply unhappy, you are prone not only to suffer from 'mental indigestion' but also from physical indigestion. Imbalances of the small intestines are characterized by holding on to things in our insides, regardless of whether these are undigested food or unresolved emotional conflicts.

It is interesting to note that the 'happiness hormone' is produced in the digestive system. In fact, 95 percent of serotonin is made in the digestive system and regulates digestive functions; only 5 percent is produced in the brain. Lack of happiness diminishes serotonin secretions and thereby weakens the digestive process.

The reverse is also true. If you are suffering from chronic indigestion or you habitually consume highly processed, refined and denatured foods, you begin to accumulate toxic waste in your intestines. This waste may give rise to nervousness, hyperactivity or any other emotionally volatile condition.

Let me put it this way. We can broadly say that toxins in the intestines are the physical counterparts of negative thoughts. And through the mind-body connection, negative thoughts and feelings translate into poisons and vice versa.

Lymph: Natural Purifier

More than two-thirds of the body's immune system is located in the intestines. And since it takes care of both physical and mental toxins, it acts as our physical and mental healing system.

Obesity, including lumpy cellulite, is one of the many conditions that results from a congested lymphatic system, which forms a large part of the body's natural immunological defenses. Other diseases include multiple sclerosis, fibromyalgia, chronic fatigue syndrome and cancer, the ultimate defense against toxins.

But what exactly is the lymphatic system? Imagine a network of drains flowing through your internal organs, taking away toxins from your tissues, blood and cells.

The drainage system is filled with fluid containing cells that transport, attack and destroy poisons such as metabolic waste, undigested food particles, animal proteins, chemicals from drugs and processed food, cellular debris, and excess fluid from the extracellular spaces or the spaces between cells.

Parts of this drainage network are located in different parts of the body including the bone marrow, thymus gland, spleen, appendix, tonsils and adenoids.

The lymph tissue in different parts of the body is connected by a network of vessels called lymph vessels. These vessels pass through purifying centers called lymph nodes that are located in the underarms, neck, chest and abdomen.

The lymph - 6 to 10 liters of lymph vis-à-vis 3.5 to 5 liters of blood - moves through the lymph nodes, which act as active purification centers. However, when the lymph fluid and immune system are overwhelmed by poisons and decomposing material from the small intestine and liver, the body loses its ability to purify itself.

Most intestinal problems occur because of eating harmful foods. The following foods or cooking processes have strongly irritating effects on the protective mucus lining present throughout the alimentary canal, from the mouth to the anus: devitalized, processed, radiated, refined, deep-fried, microwave-cooked and canned foods.

Highly acid-forming foods such as meat, fish, poultry, eggs, cheese, refined sugar, table salt, chocolate, candy, commercial fruit juices, coffee, alcohol, carbonated beverages and oral hallucinogenic and pharmaceutical drugs also irritate the intestinal lining.

Since the body cannot digest and utilize anything that is potentially harmful, these products undergo biochemical transformations, known as fermentation and putrefaction.

Studies have indicated that processed and refined foods along with alcohol and red and processed meats are a lethal combination. Not only does a diet rich in these foods promote lymph congestion and obesity over a period of time, it is also associated with an increased risk for many types of cancer - including breast, colon and pancreatic cancer.

These foods are highly acidic and have an excess of 'fire energy'. Conventional Western nutritionists call these foods 'heaty', while Chinese and other forms of natural medicine, believe they produce an excess of 'fire' energy.

Think for a moment about the metabolism of an overweight individual. Excess weight raises the body's temperature, not because the extra fat traps heat but because body's organs needs to work harder to adjust to the weight.

Even at rest, an overweight individual generates more heat than a body of normal weight. If you have a tendency towards being overweight, eating foods that are high in 'fire energy' could be a recipe for obesity and digestive problems.

Even in individuals who are not overweight, regular exposure of the intestinal lining or our 'internal skin' to acidifying and irritating components as the phosphoric acid and other chemical additives contained in colas, for example, can lead to suppurating wounds and the perforation of the intestinal walls.

Did you know that waste products from undigested food can linger in the intestinal tract for weeks, months and even years? Food that is eaten either too quickly, in between meals, late at night, or wrongly combined, lowers Agni, the digestive fire. Anger and fear also lower Agni.In an unhealthy intestinal tract, mucus, toxins and fecal matter combine to create what Ayurveda calls Ama or mucoid fecal matter. The intestines begin to lose their natural shape as they try to accommodate the extra waste. Left with no other choice, they create protrusions that are filled with layers of obstructive Ama.

Ama is a breeding ground for parasites and microbes, as well as for cancer cells. Eventually, the intestinal immune system succumbs to the overload of toxins.

Deadly microbes or harmful bacteria that are normally kept in check by the probiotic or 'good' bacteria begin to take over the digestive tract. These microbes quite literally turn everything they find into poison.

Not surprisingly, a badly congested lymphatic system leads to swelling of the abdomen and congestion in other parts of the body. In a desperate attempt to prevent the blood from being poisoned, the body begins to harden the afflicted tissue. This is the first stage of ulcerative processes.

Later, layers of hardened mucus are added, forming a thick crust around the afflicted areas. This creates further rigidity of the intestinal tract, which in turn begins to obstruct blood circulation in the intestinal wall slows down intestinal motion.

Eventually, when the immune system is completely overwhelmed, the body suffers from a toxicity crisis. Obesity is nothing but a toxicity crisis. Any attempt to reverse these destructive processes that have virtually taken over requires the body to undergo a process of detoxification. *(See Chapter 10: Coming Clean)*

Obesity and cancer are both linked to severe lymph congestion, and over the years, more and more studies have been cropping up strengthening the correlation between the two diseases.

One such study, by scientists of the University of Geneva, found a connection between obesity and tumors in the breast. The sample consisted of women diagnosed with invasive breast cancer in Geneva between 2003 and 2005.

The scientists found that the women who were obese were more likely to suffer from Stage III and Stage IV tumors with an odds ratio of 1.8. In other words, they were 180 percent more likely to develop serious breast cancer than the women who were not overweight.

Also, the obese women in the sample were 510 percent more likely to have cancerous lymph nodes, suggesting that the cancer may have spread to other parts of their bodies.

Other researchers suspect that the hormone leptin could be a 'missing link' between obesity and cancer. Leptin, produced in fat cells in adipose tissue, is also known as the satiety hormone *(See Chapter 11:* Hour of Reckoning), which tells an individual when to stop eating.

But this is not all that leptin does. This hormone is also involved in many other biological processes in the breast, from reproduction and lactation to cell differentiation and cell proliferation.

When leptin or its receptors malfunction, they are likely to promote the development of breast tumors, some scientists say.

Colon: When the Sewer Backs Up

It may surprise you to know that an increasing number of men and women have accumulated 40 pounds or more of waste material in the colon alone.

One of the organs closely linked to obesity is the large intestine or colon, whose main purpose is to prepare the waste products of metabolism for disposal via elimination.

The colon is kept clean by an organ many think is useless! The appendix grows 'good' bacteria which counteract 'bad' bacteria. Supported by bile from the liver, this tiny organ's job is to keep the colon neat and clean.

It doesn't always succeed, mainly due to unhealthy dietary habits. One of the indicators of a bowel that is not functioning effectively is constipation or frequent stools, a common symptom among individuals who are overweight.

An overloaded colon can be recognized by an enormously extended waistline. This waste accumulation may lead to a prolapsed transverse colon, which in turn, puts a great deal of pressure on the organs of the lower abdomen, including the urinary bladder, prostate or female reproductive organs. As a result, these organs may become dislocated, which causes them further structural and functional damage.

But it could get more serious than that. A study piloted by the Michigan State University published in May 2009 in the journal *Carcinogenesis* found that being overweight could increase the risk of colon cancer. Once again, the link between the two diseases was leptin.

Researchers found that levels of leptin, which regulates metabolism and hunger, are elevated in obese individuals. It also showed that chronically elevated leptin levels also induce pre-cancerous colon cells to stimulate the production of a certain growth factor.

This increases blood supply to young malignant cells, which in turn encourages the growth of cancerous tumors.

Kidneys: Stone-Walled!

The kidneys perform one of the most delicate balancing acts in the human body - maintaining the right acid-alkaline concentration of sodium and potassium in the blood and other fluids.

While sodium is an alkaline mineral, potassium is acidic. The ratio between these two natural minerals is expressed as the pH (power of hydrogen) value and needs to be maintained within an extremely narrow range.

One of the main reasons is that every one of the 100 trillion cells in your body needs a certain specific pH value so that they can perform even their basic functions. This job is entrusted to the kidneys.

If your body's internal environment tilts towards being acidic, you run the risk of suffering from acidosis, and depending on your diet, you will speed towards a toxicity crisis. Alternatively, if your blood and other fluids tilt towards being too alkaline, you run the risk of alkalosis.

When the optimal pH value is under threat, the kidneys are forced to take defensive action in an attempt to restore the imbalance. Among these measures are kidney congestion, kidney stones and fluid retention, all of which are associated with weight gain.

As we have seen with other organs such as the liver, small intestine and bowels, congestion causes a toxicity crisis, which in turn leads to various health issues such as obesity, diabetes, rheumatoid arthritis, stomach ulcers, hypertension, cancer, multiple sclerosis, Alzheimer's, and many other chronic diseases.

Some of the main factors contributing to toxicity and kidney congestion are dehydration and the consumption of acid-forming foods.

Dehydration results from insufficient water intake; consuming foods and beverages that have a dehydrating effect (meat, artificial sweeteners, sugar, alcohol, tea, coffee and sodas); smoking cigarettes; or watching television for too many hours at a stretch.

Feeding off a diet rich in acid-forming foods, such as meat, fish, dairy products, baked goods, candy, and sugar, is another way the kidneys get congested, as is consuming food and beverages that contain large amounts of oxalic acid.

Body drought occurs when you don't drink enough water. Most individuals substitute this life-giving fluid with processed beverages and drinks with caffeine such as tea and coffee.

When the body is dehydrated, the pH value gets altered. Also, the amount of water outside the cells increases to help neutralize the toxic waste products that have accumulated there.

The kidneys begin to hold on to water, drastically reducing urinary secretion and causing further retention of potentially harmful waste products.

As a result, fluid builds up in various parts of the body, selectively in some individuals and across tissues and organs in others. This puffiness and bloating, also called water edema, leads to weight gain.

If water retention alone does not actually make an individual obese, it is usually a contributory factor, more in some individuals than others.

Normally, cellular enzymes signal to the brain when cells run low on water. Enzymes in dehydrated cells, however, become so inefficient that they are no longer able to register the drought-like condition.

Subsequently, they fail to convey the emergency situation to the brain, which would normally push the 'thirst alarm button'. This results in a vicious cycle.

At the neurotransmitter level, the Renin-Angiotensin (RA) system is activated whenever there is a water shortage in the body. Apart from signaling the kidneys to inhibit urination, it also signals the blood vessels to constrict to reduce the amount of fluid circulating, which could potentially cause water loss.

This is one reason why obesity is usually accompanied by cardiovascular diseases such as hypertension.

The RA system also stimulates an increase in the absorption of sodium or salt, which helps the body retain water.

Ironic as it may sound, the main solution for water retention is to drink water! That's because it facilitates the release of toxins and brings down the acid levels in the blood and other fluids. The body no longer needs to store water to save itself. Here's something you might want to think about if you're not drinking sufficient water:

- An estimated 75 percent of Americans are chronically dehydrated
- In 37 percent of Americans, the thirst mechanism is so weak, it is mistaken for hunger. According to research at the University of Washington, drinking just one glass of water shuts down midnight hunger for almost 100 percent of dieters involved in the study
- Even mild dehydration slows down your metabolism by 3 percent.

Kidney stones are another manifestation of congestion. There are different kinds of stones depending on their composition, which in turn depends on the specific biochemical process that is off-balance.

Stones begin as tiny crystals and can eventually become as large as an egg. The tiny crystals are too small to be detected by X-rays, and since they do not cause pain, they are rarely noticed.

Yet they are big enough to block the flow of liquid through the tiny kidney tubules. Crystals or stones are formed in the kidneys when urinary constituents, which are normally in solution, are precipitated.

Precipitation occurs when these particles occur in excessive amounts or when urine becomes too concentrated. Most crystals or stones originate in the kidneys, although some may also be formed in the bladder.

If a large stone enters one of the two ureters, urinary discharge becomes obstructed. This can lead to serious complications such as kidney infection or failure.

Regardless of where in the kidneys the blockage occurs, it restricts their ability to remove and regulate water and chemicals, causing these delicate organs to suffer injury.

Some studies claim that kidney stones bring around 2 million individuals to a doctor's clinic every year. According to these studies, obese women have a 90 percent higher risk of developing kidney stones than women who are not obese. Obese men have a 33 percent higher risk.

Some researchers believe that abnormal accumulation of fat tissue induces insulin resistance, causing changes to the urine that favor the growth of kidney stones.

Others believe that another reason why obese individuals are prone to developing kidney stones is the over-consumption of soft drinks and colas.

Soft drinks are highly acidic and have radical mineral imbalances. To counterbalance this and restore the body's pH level, the kidneys draw calcium from the bones and other tissues.

Excess levels of calcium in the kidneys promote the development of stones in these organs.

Cutting soft drinks out of your diet is one of the biggest favors you can do yourself. This includes sports drinks or 'energy drinks', which according to a study by the University of Californian in Berkeley can raise body weight by a stunning 13 pounds a year if only one 20-ounce bottle is consumed every day.

Another study, conducted at Boston University School of Medicine, shows that drinking as little as one can of soda per day - regular or diet - is associated with a 46 percent increased risk of metabolic syndrome, which plays a major role in heart disease, diabetes and obesity.

According to the study, other harmful side effects of soda, both diet and regular, include:

- A 31percent greater risk of becoming obese
- A 30 percent higher risk of having a larger waistline

- A 25 percent higher risk of developing high blood triglycerides or high blood sugar
- A 32 percent greater risk of having low levels of good cholesterol
- An increased risk of high blood pressure

Chapter 4: The Big Three

People started gaining weight ever since life became more and more convenient. When modern amenities were introduced, life became sedentary and we simply got less exercise. But that's stating the obvious, isn't it?

Unfortunately, it is much more subtle than that. While a 'fatty' or sedentary lifestyle directly contributes to weight gain, the enemy is subtler than sheer laziness.

Modern conveniences often come wrapped in toxins, both literally and metaphorically. They're everywhere: in tap water, bottled water, bottled drinks, product packaging, the hundreds of chemical additives in processed foods and beverages, medical drugs, harmful low-grade radiation, and even the paint in toxic toys.

Toxins enter our bloodstream from the air we breathe, pesticides in fruit and vegetables, abnormally high levels of antibiotics and hormones in the meat of cattle, and chemical waste ingested by the fish we eat.

It is not possible to be free of toxins; neither do we need to be. A healthy body is designed to handle moderate amounts of toxic agents. However, most of us choose to live toxic lifestyles or are exposed to dangerous toxins without really being aware of it. And the human body was never meant to process the levels of toxins it is now subjected to.

The developed world is suffering from a toxicity crisis and we're paying a very heavy price. But how is a toxic lifestyle linked to being overweight?

Unholy Triad

Researchers are calling it the unholy triad. I call it The Big Three - the link between toxicity, cancer and obesity - a connection that is still at the cutting edge of medical research.

The root of obesity often leads to an organ of your body you are least likely to associate with fat - the liver. The liver is the second-largest organ of the body, after the skin, and is responsible for - hold your breath - more than 500 functions.

Before we discuss the details, let me make the connection between toxicity and obesity. The body is an extremely complex yet wonderfully synchronized machine, and an imbalance in one area may impact on an organ or a set of tissues that seem unrelated.

Toxic chemicals and other poisonous compounds may affect organs and systems without always leading to weight gain. Hence, not everyone exposed to a high degree of toxicity is overweight.

When they enter the bloodstream, poisons are stored in weak and vulnerable organs and tissues because they cannot fight back. The weakened organ becomes weaker, damaged, and diseased and eventually begins to malfunction.

This results in conditions ranging from cysts, insulin resistance, metabolic disorders, lung disease, kidney diseases, gall stones, immunological disorders (65 percent of your immune system is located in your intestines), chronic inflammation, hormonal imbalances, to cancer.

But the reverse is always true. Overweight and obese individuals are necessarily suffering from a 'toxicity crisis', a state where the body cannot handle the toxic overload.

So how does it work? Fat tissue is basically used as a safe-house for toxins. It is your body's way of keeping excess metabolic waste and other toxins out of harm's way. Storing them in fat cells, which have a low metabolic rate, keeps poisons out of the bloodstream so that they don't reach other tissues and organs.

There is no doubt that individuals who are obese harbor a severely toxic and polluted internal environment. This leads to congestion of other organs and systems. Consequently, the entire body slows down and begins to malfunction.

Have you ever wondered why some people find it difficult to lose weight? After shedding those initial extra pounds, the fat just doesn't seem to budge!

This is because a toxically overloaded system, or morbidly obese body, causes all your organs to become sluggish. As they begin to lose their natural ability to function as they were meant to, they also lose their ability to metabolize and process fat effectively.

This also makes it easier to understand why individuals who are overweight suffer from a host of health issues and diseases. There's a river of toxins - chemicals introduced to the body as well as those produced by the body in reaction to external pollutants - constantly circulating in the blood, tissues and organs.

This ultimately kick starts a vicious cycle, where toxic overload leads to obesity, and excessive fat and cellulite build-up blocks metabolism, which leads to further weight gain.

One type of toxic chemical pollutant in particular merits mention in the context of weight gain because of its notoriety. It is a group of substances called organochlorines which are used in pesticides.

Organochlorines enter the body when we eat plants sprayed with insecticides that contain these substances - DDT was banned in the US a long time ago but several other organochlorines are still widely used - and by eating animal products that contain them as cattle feed.

The problem is that organochlorines are difficult to break down and are easily attracted to fat and stored in fat cells, where they can remain for several years. If the levels of organochlorines in your body are very high, you are likely to store fat so that it can safely hide away the toxins. No wonder obese bodies are very reluctant to letting go and losing weight.

Traditional slimming techniques gauge weight loss reducing calorific intake and increasing the body's metabolic rate. This ranges from crash diets to tweaking dietary habits. It also involves rigorous exercise regimens that simultaneously burn fat quickly.

However, a vast majority of individuals also regain the weight they lose, unless they continue with stringent weight-reduction exercise programs. This ultimately exhausts and wears out the body as you are constantly working against its tendency to gain weight!

A holistic approach, on the other hand, recommends cleansing and detoxification (*See Chapter 10:* Coming Clean) of the body. This process removes years of toxic build-up and gradually repairs and restores the organs to their optimal level of functioning.

When this happens, the body also returns to its normal weight.

Liver: Natural Filter

Let me return to where it all starts - the liver. This organ is so vital to your health that it is the only organ in the body that can regenerate itself. When damaged, some individuals can manage with as little as 20 percent of their liver functioning!

Among its amazing range of functions, your liver is the main organ responsible for breaking down fat. It does this by manufacturing chemicals and enzymes that burn fat.

This organ plays a critical role in digestion by producing bile. Liver bile (it produces 1 to 1.5 quarts a day), is stored in the gall bladder and when released into the small intestine, it breaks down and digests fatty acids.

It also digests fat-soluble vitamins A, D, E and K so that they can be absorbed by the digestive tract and released into the bloodstream.

The liver is also a storage facility for metabolized food. It stores significant quantities of starch and converts it into glycogen when the body needs more energy. It stores proteins and converts them into amino acids when needed. It also stores a small amount of fats and vitamins.

The liver is the body's natural filter, detoxifying an average two quarts of blood per minute as it passes through this complex organ.

It does this by metabolizing and breaking down harmful chemicals such as ammonia, metabolic waste, drugs, and alcohol so that they, along with cellular debris, harmful microorganisms and other metabolic waste, can be eliminated through the urine and feces.

The liver also breaks down hormones that need to be eliminated from the body after they are used. Some of these hormones play a major role in various biochemical processes, such as insulin, estrogen and adrenaline. If kept in circulation, 'second-hand' hormones can be harmful for the body.

In the context of weight loss or weight gain, the liver performs three critical roles - it stores food and converts it into energy when needed; it is the body's natural filter and defense against toxins; and like a furnace, it is your body's main fat burner.

Not surprisingly, a majority of individuals who are overweight have damaged livers.

After you eat a meal and your food is digested in the small intestine, the blood from the digestive system and colon drains into the liver via the hepatic portal vein. This blood contains all the nutrients and toxins that are absorbed by the digestive tract. These nutrients are needed to feed the cells, tissues and organs of the body.

But before they can be released for circulation to various parts of the body, the blood is routed through the liver via the portal vein. The main purpose of this diversion is filtration and detoxification.

Portal hypertension, often caused by an overload of poisons and toxins, is a condition where the portal vein hardens and narrows. This leads to a vicious cycle as this condition further reduces the liver's capacity to effectively filter blood.

A toxic liver and portal hypertension affects many organs, including the bladder, colon, kidneys, rectum, and even the uterus, ovaries and Fallopian tubes.

The systems and processes of digestion and elimination are intimately and directly connected to the liver. When food is not properly digested in the small intestine, the undigested food releases poisons.

The digestive system generates toxins when we eat and drink unhealthy processed and refined foods and beverages. It also generates toxins when we use refined oil for cooking. Poisons also build up when the small intestine and liver release insufficient digestive enzymes, which causes malabsorption and malnutrition.

The colon, on the other hand, is responsible for the elimination of solid waste as feces. It may hold back undigested food and waste when it malfunctions.

This spoiling, rotting waste from the colon, along with undigested toxins from the small intestine, pours into the liver through the portal vein and poisons the organ.

When overloaded, the liver is unable to neutralize these acidic poisons and they exit the organ and enter the heart. From here, they are circulated all over the body, where they are stored in the joints, muscles, nerves, glands, brain and other vital organs.

Alternatively, when the liver is clogged with toxins, damaged, hardened and swollen, the portal vein is unable to allow the passage of blood and toxins into the liver.

The blood then backs up into various source organs, which become swollen and enlarged. Eventually, all the glands, muscles, joints and other tissues in your body become congested.

Liver: Nature's Furnace

Having established the role of the liver as a natural filter and illustrating how it is connected with digestion and elimination, let us examine the liver's role in fat metabolism.

Weight gain and weight reduction are associated with various organs and processes in the body, such as sleep cycles, hormonal balance, the immune system, and the hypothalamus which is responsible for energy regulation.

But the liver performs more fat-regulation functions than any other single organ or system alone. So just how does the liver burn or metabolize fat?

The liver regulates fat metabolism by a series of complex biochemical reactions involving hormones, natural chemicals and enzymes that act on fat.

This 'fat' includes fatty acids ingested in the food we eat, as well as fat stored in the adipose tissue that is metabolized when energy levels fall.

Fat stored under the skin and in other parts of the body is also burned when we exercise. Heightened energy oxidizes the fat but it also requires the liver to release certain hormones and enzymes to break down these fat cells. This process involves the thyroid gland as well.

Fat accumulates in the liver, gut and other parts of the body when one or more of several liver processes malfunction. One of these processes is called entero-hepatic circulation.

This is a process whereby bile acids released by the liver enter the small intestine and then make their way back to the liver along with other fluids. This circulatory process takes place several times a day through the portal vein.

Bile acids and bile salts digest dietary fat. Some of this is absorbed into the bloodstream. Fats that are not broken down by bile acids are reabsorbed by the liver from the gut and accumulate in this organ.

When you eat sufficient natural dietary fiber, excess fat as well as toxins are eliminated via the colon. However, if the fluid that re-circulates between the gut and liver is high in fats, it invariably leads to weight gain.

Also, if your liver is not functioning adequately and your gut is choked and clogged with undigested waste, it hampers the transportation of fat digested in the small intestine through the bloodstream to organs and tissues that need it.

These fats are wrapped in chylomicrons, a lipoprotein made by the small intestine. After the fat is deposited where it is needed, the remnants of chylomicrons are transported to the liver where they are processed.

If the liver is compromised by toxins, chylomicrons or fat globules cannot be absorbed by the liver and they keep circulating in the blood. These globules build up in the blood and are stored as cellulite and fat in the blood vessels, and in various body parts such as the arms, legs and midriff.

Is it any wonder then that one of the first signs of weight gain is an expanding waistline, also called 'belly fat'?

Also, a malfunctioning liver cannot manufacture sufficient high-density lipoprotein (HDL), which is needed to neutralize low-density lipoprotein (LDL) from the blood vessel walls.

So although it may not be easily apparent, a malfunctioning liver contributes to cardiovascular disease, heart disease, hypertension, atherosclerosis and makes you plain fat!

A more serious liver condition is called a 'fatty liver' or a Non-Alcoholic Liver Disease. This is a condition where excess toxins and fat build up in the liver cells and prevent the organ from, among other things, burning fat and eliminating toxins.

The liver turns into a space where fat is stored, not a furnace that burns it. A fatty liver is enlarged, greasy and gives you a pot belly. It is estimated that 20 percent of the American population has a fatty liver, with the incidence being much higher among overweight and obese individuals.

Also, though the incidence of a fatty liver is higher among individuals aged over 30, many young people including adolescents are showing signs of developing this condition.

One of the major factors contributing to a fatty liver is the consumption of processed foods which are high on chemical additives and refined sugar present in high-fructose corn syrup and refined carbohydrates.

High levels of refined sugar directly lead to a build-up of fat in the liver and also damage the mitochondria of the body's cells. Mitochondria are present in all the body's cells and, among other things, serve as 'cellular power plants' because they generate most of the cell's supply of chemical energy.

When mitochondria are damaged, cellular energy drops, which slows down metabolism; and slower metabolism naturally means weight gain and reduced energy.

Having established the overwhelming connection between toxicity and the liver, let us complete the unholy triad and make the connection between these two conditions and cancer.

Cancer: Toxic Cells

Cancer, like any other so-called disease, does not develop overnight. It is the result of several crises of toxicity whose root cause is one or more energy-depleting influences.

Stimulants, emotional trauma, repressed feelings, irregular lifestyle, dehydration, nutritional deficiency, overeating, chronic stress, lack of sleep, and the accumulation of heavy metals thwart the body's efforts to remove metabolic waste, poisons and the debris of 30 billion cells that die naturally every day.

When these poisons accumulate in any part of the body, they lead to a number of progressive healing responses that include irritation, swelling, hardening, inflammation, ulceration and even abnormal growth of cells.

Like every other disease, cancer is a toxicity crisis and it marks the body's final attempt to rid itself of septic poisons and acidic compounds that result from not being able to effectively remove metabolic waste, toxins and putrefying dead cells in the body.

It may surprise you to read this but cancer is the body's last-ditch attempt to save itself. It is an attempt at self-preservation. (You can read more about this in my books *Cancer is Not a Disease* and *Timeless Secrets of Health and Rejuvenation*)

And herein lies the link between cancer and obesity - toxicity. Is it pure coincidence that apart from other diseases, individuals who are obese are at a higher risk of cancer than those who are not?

This is an undisputable fact supported by years of painstaking research. It is also no coincidence that obesity is closely related to heart disease and diabetes, two other major illnesses that are the result of overloading the body with external and internal toxins, and that are often triggered by emotional trauma or conflict.

Cells only go into a defensive mode and turn malignant (become mal-aligned) if they need to ensure their own survival. A spontaneous remission occurs when cells no longer need to defend themselves. Hence, when the crisis comes to a resolution and the body feels no longer threatened, it will start healing and repairing itself. During the healing and repair phase, the tumor will become inflamed and enlarged before it is finally broken down by 'infectious' bacteria and fungi. As research has shown, every spontaneous remission is accompanied by an infection and fever. If the healing phase becomes intercepted through the use of radiation, chemotherapy, surgery, anti-inflammatory drugs and or antibiotics, the spontaneous remission does not occur and the need for secondary tumors may arise in the future.

With the correct approach, though, a tumor as big as an egg can spontaneously regress and disappear, regardless of whether it is in the brain, the stomach, breast or ovary. I have seen a bladder tumor as large as an orange on a live ultrasound picture collapse into itself and disintegrate within 15 seconds. As always, the tumor fragments end up coming out with the urine. This should not be considered a miracle, but just the normal, natural way of the body returning to homeostasis. The cure phase begins when the toxicity crisis stops. The disease symptoms merely indicate that the body is actively healing and repairing itself. Feeling really bad during this phase actually shows the body is profoundly engaged in healing itself.

A toxicity crisis ends when we cease to deplete the body's energy and remove existing toxins from the blood, bile ducts, lymph ducts and cell tissues. Unless the body has been seriously damaged by interfering programs, it is perfectly capable of taking care of the rest, without much discomfort.

Medical intervention, on the other hand, reduces the possibility of a spontaneous remission to almost zero because of its suppressive and debilitating effects. Just the diagnosis of cancer, which serves as a death threat, is one the most stressful events a human being can experience. It starts off a series of powerful stress responses that biologically suppresses or deactivates the most vital functions in the body, such as digestion, sleep, metabolism, and waste removal. Hence, under prolonged stress, the cells become undernourished, lymph and blood flow turns sluggish, and the body loses weight and strength. Any treatment that follows the cancer diagnosis further increases the death fright, especially if it drains the patient of every ounce of energy he has left.

Of course, all this prevents the body from going through the natural healing and repair cycles that I discusssed before. If the patient dies, the doctors blame the cancer for it, whereas in truth, it is the diagnosis and the treatment that are responsible for the wasting and severe decline of the vital functions of the body. A cancer is part of the body healing response, not its killer. Although a tumor mass may become temporarily obstructive, it rarely does any harm.

Of the 30 billion cells that a healthy body turns over each day, at least 1 percent are cancer cells. Does this mean that all of us are destined to develop cancer - the disease? Certainly not.

These cancer cells are products of 'programmed mutation' that keep the immune system alert, active and stimulated. So why does cancer manifest itself in different tissues and organs in different people? Why do some toxic individuals develop cardiovascular disease while others put on weight while still others develop cancer?

The answer lies in the complex and dynamic interplay of psychological, physiological and biochemical processes in the body and the unique ways in which they are present in each one of us.

Disease manifests itself in organs that are weak, which are the most vulnerable to poisons. Each organ reacts differently. Hence, different types of diseases show up in different individuals but each one is the manifestation of a toxicity crisis, which typically also includes a social/emotional conflict.

Cancer cells are cells that are, over time, deprived of oxygen and nutrients due to the gradual build up of congestion in the intercellular fluids. To compensate the diminished biological capacity of the affected organ, the body begins to produce extra cells. The new cells are specially marked so that the body can identify and destroy them again once the crisis has passed. The body even creates new blood vessels to support these important cells during the crisis. A cancerous tumor is born once the toxicity crisis has reached its peak and the healing can begin.

During the healing phase, when the extra cells are no longer needed to sustain the body during the survival crisis, the tumor will swell, become inflamed and cause pain. At the final stage of the tumor growth, specialized destructive bacteria and fungi start the decomposition process and the tumor breaks up, provided no painkillers or antibiotics are used to stop this process. This is the natural progression and end of any cancer.

There is another connection between obesity and cancer, one that is again largely ignored by medical science - the emotional aspect. Constant conflicts, guilt and shame, for example, can easily paralyze the body's most basic functions, and lead to the growth of a cancerous tumor. I want to emphasize again that cancer cells are specialized emergency cells that support us during a stressful, difficult time. Once we are back to a relaxed, settled state in our body and mind, the body will deliver special immune cells, fluids, and micro-organisms to the site of these helper cells. The tumor that is being formed during this healing process is the body's natural method of doing away with the now unnecessary emergency cells.

Cancer cannot occur unless there has been a strong undercurrent of emotional uneasiness and deep-seated frustration some time prior to its appearance. Cancer patients typically suffer from lack of self-respect or worthlessness, and often have what I call an 'unfinished business' or 'unresolved conflict' in their life. Also infants who are born prematurely or otherwise experience a separation conflict when they are not breastfed or allowed to be with their mother most of the time during the first few months or years of their life, or are injected with poison-filled vaccines, can easily develop cancer as a coping mechanism. Cancer cells are cells that help us survive in a 'hostile', toxic environment. In other words, like obesity, cancer is as much a natural reaction to emotional toxins as it is a defense against a chemical assault.

Letting go of the need to fight in life reprograms the body's DNA, changing its course of warfare and eventual annihilation to one of healthy reproduction. The fear of cancer is deeply ingrained in our society's collective beliefs. It is worsened by the doom and gloom approaches of modern medicine. Obesity, cancer, and any other 'disease' is not something we need to be afraid of. Knowledge is power. Knowing that the body never makes mistakes also removes the fear of disease. Allowing the body to go through its own healing process (mistaken for a disease), is the best you can do for yourself. The recognition that obesity is a protective mechanism that actually saves your life can provide you with enough motivation to truly take care of your body just like you would take care of your own child.

Pumping Poisons

Xenoestrogens: High levels of toxicity, the rising incidence of obesity and cancer are all ailments of modern life that have become health issues over the last four decades.

If you are looking for a physical link between obesity and cancer, here it is. Medical science has found that both fatty tissues in obese individuals as well as cancerous tumors, in general, reveal a high level of toxins and poisons stored in them.

One group of these toxins is a class of compounds called xenoestrogens, synthetic compounds so-called because they mimic the female hormone estrogen.

Xenoestrogens are present in a wide range of industrial and agricultural chemicals such as plastics and pesticides and they tend to 'estrogenize' the environment depending on where you live and the types of products you use.

Take the simple plastic bottle or yoghurt container, for example. Among the chemicals in these polycarbonate plastics are bisphenol A and phthalates, which are believed to be carcinogenic. They specifically target the prostate gland in men.

From here, it is not difficult to make the connection between bisphenol A and phthalates, obesity and cancer. Prostate cancer is the most common form of cancer in men. Also, obesity more than doubles the risk of prostate cancer in men. Get the connection?

Also, overweight men tend to develop more aggressive forms of prostate cancer and are at higher risk of recurrence and metastasis (when cancer spreads).

Studies have also demonstrated a connection between low sperm counts in men and their fetal exposure to xenoestrogens through their mothers.

But women are not spared. These carcinogenic chemical compounds also place women at risk. They are believed to disrupt the female reproductive system as well as increase the risk of breast cancer.

To get an idea of just how versatile xenoestrogens are, read this list: atrazine (weed killer), 4-Methylbenzylidene camphor (4-MBCin sunscreen lotions, butylated hydroxyanisole (BHA in food preservative), bisphenol A (monomer for polycarbonate plastic and epoxy resin, antioxidant in plasticizers), dichlorodiphenyldichloroethylene (one of the breakdown products of DDT), dieldrin (insecticide), DDT (insecticide), endosulfan (insecticide), erythrosine (FD&C Red No 3), heptachlor (insecticide), lindane (hexachlorocyclohexane in insecticide), metalloestrogens (a class of inorganic xenoestrogens), methoxychlor (insecticide), nonylphenol and derivatives (industrial surfactants, emulsifiers for emulsion polymerization, laboratory detergents, pesticides), pentachlorophenol (general biocide and wood preservative), polychlorinated biphenyls (PCBs in electrical oils, lubricants, adhesives, paints), parabens (lotions), phenosulfothiazine (a red dye), phthalates (plasticizers) and DEHP (plasticizer for PVC).

What does this mean in everyday language? It means these toxic and carcinogenic chemicals are lurking in more places than you probably imagine.

Xenoestrogens are an ingredient in DDT, a powerful pesticide now banned in the US. But vegetables imported from countries where this pesticide is liberally used pose a serious toxic risk.

DDT metabolizes in the body into a substance called DDE, which is xenoestrogenic and remains in the body for several years.

Xenoestrogens are also found in plastic containers used to store large quantities of water, in detergents, spermicides, personal care products, and plastics used to package food.

Sometimes, these compounds may be closer home than you think. A group of researchers at Dartmouth University is reported to have found them in the plastic wrap of food products. Others have found them in the coating in metal cans, food containers, refrigerator shelving, baby bottles, microwave ovenware, and utensils used to eat.

Biologists have found that fish that breed in water that is highly contaminated with sewage and other pollutants show sexual characteristics of both sexes. These sexually confused fish tested positive for high levels of xenoestrogens.

More bad news. Livestock raised on cattle farms in some countries are administered xenoestrogens, which causes water-retention and 'fatten' them up quickly at low cost. Cattle farmers reap fat profits but consumers are placed at considerable health risk.

Cosmetics and beauty products are another rich source of carcinogenic products. Breast tumors have shown high levels of parabens, a type of xenoestrogen in deodorants, antiperspirants, skin lotions, gels and shampoos.

Here is another alarming finding. Many popular sunscreen lotions contain xenoestrogens, which have been linked to endometriosis. About 5 to 10 percent of women in the US are affected by endometriosis, which is known to induce infertility. Put two and two together (including exposure to xenoestrogens from other sources) and it is not hard to make the connection.

While looking for a further correlation between obesity and cancer, researchers discovered the following. The liver, a powerful organ of detoxification, usually metabolizes and thus removes two estrogen compounds from the body during the last stages of ovulation, which occurs prior to the next menstrual cycle. These are estradiol and estrone.

If the liver is already congested with toxins and other waste, as it is in obese women, the organ fails to remove these used hormones from the bloodstream. Hence their levels remain high in the blood.

However, in their used-up form, these hormonal products are toxic to the body's tissues and cause what women usually refer to as Pre-Menstrual Syndrome or PMS: breast tenderness, pain, cramping, and irritability, among other things.

Estrone: Studies have demonstrated that women with higher levels of estrone are also at a higher risk for reproductive tissue cancers including breast cancer. Obese women also have higher levels of estrone, and are also at a higher risk for PMS. This further strengthens the obesity-cancer link.

Oxidative Stress: According to a November 2009 report by the American Institute for Cancer Research, more than 100,000 Americans develop cancer due to obesity every year. The study claims there is a direct correlation between excess body fat and various types of cancer.

- endometrial cancer: 49 percent
- esophageal cancer: 35 percent
- pancreatic cancer: 28 percent
- kidney cancer: 24 percent
- gallbladder cancer: 21 percent
- breast cancer: 17 percent
- colorectal cancer: 9 percent

The study pointed out that excess body fat stimulates the secretion of certain hormones and sex steroids that promote cancer growth.

Many other studies too have found a strong correlation between obesity and cancer. In line with earlier findings, this study links cancer to two factors, one of them being toxicity (explained above), and the other being oxidative stress.

As far as toxicity is concerned, we have already established that adipose tissue is a safe-house for storing poisons and various harmful chemicals that would unleash havoc if they were released into the bloodstream.

Toxins are by nature acidic waste. When the body is overwhelmed by too much toxicity, it makes the blood acidic and thus threatens to tip the delicate acid-alkaline balance or pH level.

When the body can no longer maintain the required acid-alkaline balance, it has to devise a new way to defend itself. Instead of suffocating in their own waste, the DNA of the cells in our body mutate and often take the fall. They get damaged, diseased and mutate, ironically, in a desperate effort to survive. Cells with damaged DNA are predisposed to turning cancerous.

Over time, bad food choices and unhealthy dietary habits, severely alters the ability of the body to neutralize and eliminate acidic toxic waste. This is probably why obese individuals are more prone to cancer.

The second causative link between obesity and cancer is a phenomenon called oxidative stress. Excess body fat increases oxidative stress on the body, which compromises the immune system and, just like toxicity, also damages DNA. This creates an environment that is conducive to both the formation and reproduction of cancer cells.

Oxidative stress results from the damage that free radicals cause to the cells of your body. Free radicals are highly unstable, negatively charged atoms or molecules that are released by your cells during metabolism.

Your body has an in-built mechanism that normally neutralizes these potentially damaging agents with the help of enzymes and antioxidants. But when your cells produce too many free radicals, it results in oxidative damage, a process whereby these atoms or molecules attach themselves to healthy cells and damage proteins, lipids, membranes and DNA in the cells.

Oxidative damage is connected to the aging process as well as several diseases such as Alzheimer's and cancer. Environmental factors and lifestyle habits such as pollution, too much exposure to sunlight and smoking also trigger the production of free radicals.

Vitamin D & Cancer: In a new study at the forefront of research on Vitamin D and cancer, researchers at the University of California, San Diego School of Medicine and the Moores Cancer Center predicted that 75 percent of deaths from breast cancer and colorectal cancer could be prevented with adequate intake of Vitamin D3 and calcium.

This might seem like a simple solution to a complex pathological process but when you examine the logic (not to mention the growing body of research supporting the Vitamin D3-cancer link), the pieces fall in place.

The focal point of this approach - called 'Micro-Darwinian Carcinogenesis' - is the pivotal role that Vitamin D3 and calcium play in the cell junctions. These are the main nutrients needed by the microscopic but complex structures that hold cells together and prevent the body from falling apart, as it were.

These structures, or hinges or joints, form the scaffolding that make for the integrity and cohesiveness of tissue. When the scaffolding weakens, the cells begin to pull apart.

When cells act in unison, the expression of their individual characteristics is inhibited and the organ remains healthy. Deficiencies in calcium or Vitamin D3 at the cell junctions allow the cells the freedom to express their idiosyncrasies.

Should even a minute number of these cells contain damaged DNA, they will tend to reproduce aggressively and rapidly, leading to cancerous tumors that could later spread.

Researchers have found that the greater the integration and cohesiveness of cells, the greater the resistance to turning cancerous. They call this process of 'uncoupling' of cells 'disjunction'.

If this takes place in tissue with damaged DNA, the rest of the steps in the development of a cancerous tumor are likely to follow. However, researchers believe that adequate Vitamin D3 and calcium can prevent disjunction.

The Whole Truth

Everything we experience is a holistic combination of our mind, body and spirit. This simply means that when you break down every experience, each one can be classified into a thought, feeling and the life force associated with it.

The life force is the chi or positive energy that powers our every cell, keeps our organs, systems and bodies going, and directly affects our health and state of well-being.

When we are in harmony with ourselves, our body and environment, our energies flow freely, giving us a sense of well-being. It is a powerful force that usually remains in the realm of the subconscious, keeping each one of us alive and powering us on.

Different systems of thought interpret the life force differently but it boils down to vibrational energies that exist within every animate and inanimate object, and that relates every object to every other.

These energies can be either positive or negative. When there is conflict and resistance, the life force is blocked, diverted and disrupted, and this contributes to disease and ill-health. Negative energy blocks the free flow of energy through the body's energy channels or pathways.

Positive energy, on the other hand, allows our bodies to function as they are meant to - optimally and in a state of vibrant health.

This eventually translates into physical and chemical energy that acts on our cells, tissues, organs and systems.

The level on which the life force works is usually subliminal, i.e. below the threshold of consciousness. Hence we are not aware of it. But the fact remains that we are more intimately connected to ourselves and our environment than we realize. And this plays a pivotal role in our state of heath or disease including weight loss and weight gain.

Bodily processes, on the other hand, need little introduction, except to that say that they are the focus of classic systems of medicine. These systems, such as allopathy, address symptoms of disease with powerful chemical drugs, often quite efficiently.

But this view of medicine takes only half a view of the mind-body connection as it focuses only on physiological processes.

A holistic approach, on the other hand, believes that the mind and body do not exist as separate entities. Each one has a powerful influence on the other and one cannot exist without the other.

Mind-body medicine is gaining ground and even some medical practitioners are realizing the limitations of taking a telescopic view of the human condition.

How do we relate this to weight loss? Obesity is as much a state of mind as it is a physical state. I do not mean it is imagined or that you can simply wish it away. It means getting in touch with your inner self and connecting with every aspect of yourself, both conscious and unconscious.

It means relating to yourself intimately and discovering your basic beliefs and assumptions about yourself and the world in general; examining your world view and finding out how you perceive yourself in relation to other people, to your environment and to life's circumstances.

More than what you really *are*, being overweight or obese is about who you *think* you are.

Emotional Memory

This brings us to the other aspect of being human - our emotions. Many of us are virtually ruled by our emotions. They influence our every waking moment; they dictate who our friends are, our attitudes towards ourselves, other people and life in general; and they determine the important decisions we make.

Our emotions form a critical aspect of the mind-body connection and can determine whether you can successfully cleanse yourself and lose weight or whether you desperately want to hold on to excess weight as a defense mechanism.

In the earlier part of this chapter, we discussed physical toxins and how they impair our body, compromise its functioning, congest our organs and systems, and ultimately drive us to put on weight.

Let us now discuss emotional toxins and their significance in weight regulation.

An emotion starts with a thought or image in the mind - stressful, calming or exciting. Every thought and feeling is instantly translated into biochemical compounds within the brain and within every other part of the body.

Sustained emotional states therefore alter our very biochemistry and internal physiology. When they are strong enough and last long enough, they are apparent even in our physical appearance.

In fact, every bit of mental activity leaves us with a specific physical sensation, known as emotion. Emotions are composites of both mental impulses and physical changes, and they express the totality of one's health at any given time.

These biochemical processes are essentially hormonal changes. For instance, if you think of a stressful situation like an altercation you had with someone you dislike, the body reacts by releasing the stress hormones adrenaline, cortisol and cholesterol.

These hormones are released into the bloodstream in response to anger, fear or rejection. These states constitute what psychologists call the 'flight or fight' response, which is a survival mechanism.

However, if these hormones are secreted in an ongoing manner - when you are in a prolonged state of uncertainty, anxiety, fear or dejection - they could damage your blood vessels and impair your immune system.

Your happy emotions, on the other hand, manifest as endorphins, serotonin, interleukin II, among others, that relate to experiences of pleasure and satisfaction. If you produce enough of these chemicals, you may even be able to arrest the aging process.

Controlled studies have shown that you can reduce your biological age by 10 to 15 years within 10 days, provided your interpretation of your life experience undergoes rapid and radical changes. Alternatively, you can also put on 20 extra years within a single day if you enter a state of hopelessness and depression.

Hormones produce extremely powerful effects, both positive and negative. Yet even more powerful than hormones are the thoughts and intentions that trigger them.

Research has shown that all our thoughts, feelings, emotions, desires, intentions, beliefs and realizations are instantly translated into neuropeptides or neurotransmitters in the brain. These hormones are the chemical messengers of information. The messages they deliver determine how your body functions.

Scientists have already identified over a hundred neuropeptides, and many more are believed to exist. A nerve cell or neuron produces and uses these peptides to transmit information to other neurons. This form of transmission, called 'firing', takes place in each of the millions of neurons in our brain, all at the same time!

As soon as they are used, peptides are neutralized by enzymes, erasing all physical evidence of that thought or feeling. But make no mistake: the experience is stored in the memory bank of your consciousness or subconscious. If you need to, or if there is an appropriate stimulus in your environment, you will be able to recall or remember it.

This brings us to a fundamental question that is currently the subject of research and experimentation: is the brain the ultimate authority of your body? How do the millions of neurons know which type of neurotransmitter they need to make for each specific thought, at the very moment it occurs?

What causes them to 'fire' simultaneously throughout the brain and nervous system? And more stunning, how does one neuron know what the other neuron thinks when there is no direct physical connection between the two?

In recent years, scientists have discovered that these chemical messengers are not made by brain cells alone but also by all the other cells in the body. This brings us to the next question: Do we think only with our brain cells or also with other cells in the body?

There is indeed enough scientific evidence to show that skin cells, liver cells, heart cells, immune cells, etc all have the same remarkable ability to think, emote and make decisions as brain cells.

Have you ever stopped to wonder how certain phrases in the English language originated? Such as "I have a gut feeling" or adjectives such as 'bilious', 'phlegmatic' and 'sanguine', which relate to an old system of belief that temperament and personality types originated from four 'humors' in the body: yellow bile, black bile, phlegm and blood.

Whether the 'four-humors' view is accurate or not, the fact is that since time immemorial, medicine has related behavior and emotion to the physical body, and this is the crux of a holistic approach.

Some holistic practitioners also believe that specific emotional states are localized in specific organs, such as anger in the liver; fear in the kidneys, and depression in the lungs.

Imagine the implications this would have for individuals who are overweight. Not only is a toxic body railing against losing weight; the mind is also cooperating with it!

Toxic Beliefs

Individuals who are preoccupied with negative attitudes and emotions - fear, anger, resentment, unresolved conflict, jealousies, pessimism - are said to live in an emotionally toxic state.

Since we would be overwhelmed by our emotions if we experienced all of them consciously all of the time, we tend to suppress or repress them or store them away in the subconscious.

But even when these feelings and attitudes don't exist at the conscious level, the negative emotional energy remains embedded in our body's energy fields and they continue to alter our biochemistry and health.

An emotionally toxic state invariably targets the organs of elimination, simply because it is these organs that rid our bodies of chemical poisons and metabolic waste: the liver, kidneys, skin, lungs and colon.

Unresolved emotions and conflicts block the energy or life force and energy fields of these organs. When they malfunction, physical toxins build up and congest our systems and toxicity levels rise. Now emotional toxicity and physical poisons begin to work in tandem, creating a vicious cycle of toxicity and weight gain.

If you take a deep breath and reverse everything you have read in this chapter, the solution to weight gain is clear. In a nutshell, this means: As you gained, so you shall lose. (We shall discuss detoxification in a later chapter)

Classic methods of weight loss, either through dieting or exercise, push your body to its limits. They suggest that you must exert your will and summon every last ounce of energy to 'conquer' the battle of the bulge.

Weight reduction the natural way recommends gentle and gradual cleansing and detoxification. It is a process that restores your body and mind to their natural, optimal state of functioning.

Since *this* is how your body and mind were meant to be, it makes logical sense to seek equilibrium and balance, rather than punish your mind and body into an exceedingly uncomfortable space. After all, why blame your body for being overweight?

Chapter 5: Biological Warfare

On the physical level, the human body is a mass of cells that interact with each other through a complex interplay of biochemical reactions fuelled by the food we eat.

What happens when our natural biochemistry is altered, either temporarily or permanently? What is responsible for these biochemical changes? And how are they connected to weight loss or weight gain?

I shall attempt to answer these questions in this chapter, with specific focus on medical drugs, the delicate yet robust endocrine balance your body needs in order to maintain good health, and how metabolic disturbances lead to weight gain.

Drugs: Cure or Disease?

Pharmaceutical drugs are designed to treat the symptoms of various diseases. They are usually strong, they tend to remove the symptoms of disease fairly quickly, and in the case of serious illnesses, they alleviate discomfort and pain. No wonder they are so addictive!

There is another reason why most individuals reach out for allopathic drugs so nonchalantly - an unspoken pact between the billion-dollar pharma industry, doctors who wittingly or unwittingly promote them, and the media which promotes the industry's vested interests.

As a result, we tend to ignore the full impact a drug might have on our bodies, not to mention the results of so-called trials conducted by pharma companies intent on pushing these chemical formulations onto a vulnerable and ill-informed public.

Often, we are not aware that a certain drug may have undesirable and even dangerous side-effects simply because a clever media and advertising campaign may have brainwashed us into believing that a certain company may have discovered a certain 'cure'.

Remember, in Chapters 3 and 4, we examined the liver's role in weight gain? This vital organ is no longer able to effectively regulate the metabolism of fats and other fuels when its ability to detoxify harmful substances is compromised. Since the liver performs more than 500-odd functions, a sick liver usually has devastating and cascading consequences.

Along with the small intestine, the liver is at the centre of the body's digestive processes. When the liver is damaged, fatty deposits build up inside, fat accumulates elsewhere in the body as well and the systems of digestion and elimination back up and congest other tissues and organs. One of the many consequences of a damaged liver is weight gain.

In some acute conditions, you develop a 'fatty liver', where abnormal amounts of fats are stored the organ's cells and internal spaces. A clogged liver cannot break down and process poisons for elimination, leading to toxic congestion.

Alternatively, a healthy liver detoxifies harmful substances by metabolizing them. And among the wide variety of poisons it filters are chemicals released into the bloodstream by pharmaceutical drugs.

Before we look at some common drugs that interfere with the liver's functioning, let's look at the process by which the liver performs this all-important task and what could happen should something upset its ability to filter your blood.

Allopathic drugs by their very definition are xenobiotic ('foreign to a living organism') chemicals. They are manmade or synthetic and were never intended by nature to be introduced to the body.

Hence, apart from releasing chemicals that alleviate the symptoms of disease, they also release substances that harm the body.

Drugs are metabolized by the liver in the smooth tissue called the endoplasmic reticulum. This takes place in two phases. During the first phase, the liver's enzymes oxidize, reduce and hydrate the toxins.

These chemical compounds are rendered water soluble so that they can be absorbed by the bloodstream and carried to an organ or tissue they were meant to 'treat'. But this process also generates compounds called 'metabolites' that are toxic to the human body.

These metabolites are chemically neutralized by the cells of the liver in the second phase of drug metabolism. These metabolites are thus rendered inert so that they can be excreted through the urine.

But it is not as simple as that. Take, for instance, one of America's most-popular over-the-counter drugs - Tylenol (or Panadol) - and prescription drugs such as Vicodin and Percocet. These hugely popular analgesics belong to a class of drugs called acetaminophen and are the most widely used drugs to treat pain and fever in the US.

To make sure acetaminophen can be consumed by all age groups, it is available as a children's dissolvable, in chewable form, suspension form, and, of course, as tablets to be swallowed.

One of the devastating effects of too much acetaminophen is acute liver failure. This drug releases a toxic metabolite called N-acetyl-p-benzoquinone-imine NAPQI, or NABQI, which is further broken down before it is rendered harmless.

However, this toxic metabolite has an affinity for liver proteins and binds to them usually before it can be broken down and neutralized. Individuals who pop too many painkillers or pop them all too frequently are in danger of overdosing (fatal or not) on acetaminophen and sustaining hepatotoxicity (a toxic liver) and massive liver damage.

Acetaminophen is especially associated with oxidative damage and mitochondrial dysfunction. This causes major injury to the liver's cells, which makes them inflamed. The cells then begin to die. This drug can also damage the kidneys.

How often have you heard of someone dying from an overdose of painkillers?

Finally, taking note of the widespread liver damage caused by acetaminophen, the Food and Drug Administration (FDA) in June 2009 said it was examining the possible removal of acetaminophen from some popular analgesic combination products such as Vicodin. It added that it was also considering lowering the maximum daily dose (currently 4 gm in adults and 90 mg/kg in children).

The pharma industry is notorious for either not informing the public of possible side effects of the drugs they make, for not conducting all the mandatory tests and trials, or both. This coupled with a watchdog body - the FDA - that is not stringent enough.

As a result, research findings keep cropping up even years after a certain drug may have been given the go-ahead by the FDA. One such group of drugs that was only later found to induce hepatotoxicity is called Non-Steroidal Anti-Inflammatory Drugs or NSAIDs.

Among the more popular NSAIDs are aspirin, phenylbutazone (Butazoledine), sulindac (Clinoril), piroxicam (Feldene), diclofenac (Voltaren) and indomethacin (Indocin). These are generic names for many of the popular tablets and capsules we use to treat various commonly occurring diseases.

Apart from the dangers of using NSAIDs, many of these drugs also induce side effects that are idiosyncratic. This means their adverse reactions are unpredictable and can occur without warning. It is a convenient escape hatch for drug companies to stifle opposition from a vigilant public or to ward off lawsuits.

Yet another class of drugs that is widely prescribed by doctors is glucocorticoids, which act on the immune system to reduce inflammation. They also affect carbohydrate mechanism and fat formation.

Glucocorticoids tend to stimulate the appetite, increase the storage of glycogen in the liver and tend to cause what is referred to as 'central obesity' or the accumulation of fat in the abdomen and trunk.

Due to their powerful anti-inflammatory effects and ability to suppress the immune system, synthetic glucocorticoids are used to treat symptoms such as allergies, asthma, autoimmune diseases and sepsis.

For instance, Fluticasone or Flonase (nasal sprays containing glucocorticoids) are widely used to treat allergies while several lotions and gels are prescribed for the treatment of skin rashes.

We pop pills for various reasons - coughs and colds, aches and pains, and more serious ailments such as arthritis, hypertension, infections and many more. Doctors and patients (the general population) are so brainwashed into believing that chemical drugs will cure or at least alleviate our physical ailments that we tend to act in a blinkered way.

This reasoning is fundamentally flawed. One, what modern medicine leads us to believe are diseases are actually symptoms of something else - a toxicity crisis. This is the body's way of signaling that there is an imbalance in our bodies and our lifestyle that is throwing the internal environment out of balance. Even cancer, projected as a terminal illness, is not a disease (*Read more about this in my book* Cancer Is Not A Disease).

The second flawed assumption is that pharmaceutical drugs will cure these diseases. As we have just seen, synthetic chemical drugs, while appearing to alleviate or mask symptoms of illness, actually *add* to the toxicity crisis in the body.

Instead, the toxicity crisis, even in severe conditions, can be reversed through gentle and painless means discussed later in this book.

The Elusive 'Magic' Pill

Science and pharma companies have always conspired to find a 'magic pill' that can 'cure' obesity, or at least something that can be marketed as a panacea for the gullible and overweight population.

Their search for this elusive pill is no doubt driven solely by profit and not your health or well-being.

When amphetamines were given to German soldiers to tackle the food crisis during the Second World War, medical science was jubilant. Amphetamines were found to decrease hunger and the medical fraternity thought they had hit pay dirt.

After the war, amphetamines were commercially sold as an appetite suppressant in the market. They were finally banned from sale in the 1950s, when the authorities realized that they were being abused for recreational use.

Today, there is a wide variety of pills that promise to control food intake flooding the US market. And an unsuspecting and overweight population looking for an 'easy cure' is buying into the hype built around these drugs.

So if amphetamines, which are psychostimulants, were banned from commercial sale due to their addictive properties in the 1950s, they were replaced by a plethora of diet pills that now go by various names - appetite-suppressants, appetite-depressants and the less ominous sounding 'dietary supplement' or 'weight-loss supplement'.

These so-called anti-obesity drugs or 'diet pills' are called anoretics or anorexigenics. They limit or rein in food intake and therefore reduce the number of calories consumed. They diminish appetite in one of two ways.

Depending on the chemical reaction they induce, they either shrink your appetite or trick your brain into believing that you are 'full' even if your glucose levels indicate the opposite. This is called the 'satiety response'.

The logic is simple - if you eat less, you are less likely to put on weight. Better still, you will lose weight. In the rush to buy a quick-fix solution to their weight-gain problem, few overweight individuals spare a thought for the damaging and potentially dangerous effects these pills have on the body's biochemistry.

Diet pills or appetite-suppressants are synthetic drugs (we already know what they do to the liver) which trigger and manipulate hormones and neurotransmitters that regulate the body's metabolism and mood.

These include catecholamines and serotonin, norepinephrine and dopamine, which are critical neurotransmitters that affect various processes at various sites in the body.

Take sibutramine (brand name Meridia in the US and Reductil in Europe), for instance. This drug, a short-term appetite-suppressant, works by acting on serotonin, dopamine and norepinephrine, all of them neurotransmitters.

But the drug has run into controversy, with reports of heart failure, renal failure, gastrointestinal problems and even death associated with it.

Following a public outcry against appetite suppressants, the FDA issued an alert in December 2008, naming 27 products marketed as 'dietary supplements' for weight loss that illegally contain sibutramine.

In March 2009, there were reports that certain Chinese 'herbal supplements' sold in Europe contained twice the dosage of the licensed version of the drug. That is not all. In April 2009, the FDA banned 34 more 'herbal supplements' from the market, taking the total to 72 'diet pills' and other weight-loss products tainted with hidden and dangerous drugs and chemicals. Most of these are being imported from China.

The most commonly found chemicals in these formulations are: sibutramine (controlled substance), phenytoin (anti-seizure medication), phenolphthalein (solution used in chemical experiments and a possible carcinogen) and bumetanide (diuretic).

Following are some more chemicals you would be surprised to find in 'diet pills': Fenproporex (a stimulant not approved for marketing in the US that can cause high blood pressure, palpitations, arrhythmia), fluoxetine (active ingredient in Prozac, a prescription antidepressant), furosemide (active ingredient in Lasix, a potent diuretic that can cause severe dehydration and electrolyte imbalance), and rimonabant (active ingredient in Zimulti, not approved in the US due to increased risk of neurological and psychiatric side-effects).

Many of the products that contain these chemicals masquerade as 'natural' or 'herbal' formulations, and with very good reason. Dietary supplements were originally meant to be herbal remedies that do not need FDA approval as they are made from natural herbs, plants, seeds and even chitin, a starch found in the skeleton of shrimp, crab and other shellfish.

But the fact is that most of these so-called herbal formulations illegally contain synthetic chemicals, which make them 'more effective' but which have devastating consequences on your health.

This is an unregulated market with little or no controls. Considering the millions of dollars at stake and the competition driving the market, many of these so-called herbal magic potions sold over the counter are actually dangerous toxic cocktails.

Why, some over-the-counter weight-loss drugs work by using an anesthetic called benzocaine to numb the mouth and make eating distasteful! Yes, people are actually buying it.

Let us now a look at a weight-loss prescription drug that is not an appetite-suppressant but a 'lipase inhibitor'. Generically called orlistat (brand name Xenical), this chemical was approved by the FDA in 1999 for weight regulation. This is, in fact, one of the few weight-loss drugs approved for use for at least 12 months at a time.

What orlistat does is it blocks the enzymes in the small intestine from metabolizing fats ingested in your food into smaller molecules that can be absorbed by the body. This drug is believed to thwart the body's ability to digest fats by as much as one-third, thus promoting weight loss.

What happens to the fat that is not absorbed? The makers of the drug claim it is eliminated through feces. Indeed, orlistat produces oily stools. But in June 2009, orlistat made its way to the FDA's list of drugs that are under investigation for potential safety issues, in this case, liver toxicity, gallstones, kidney stones, abnormal blood thinning and precancerous colon lesions.

The FDA's move followed a public interest campaign mounted by consumer groups in 2006, as soon as GlaxoSmithKline received conditional approval from the FDA to sell Xenical over the counter in a half-strength tablet called Alli.

Diet pills have a controversial record, with several of them being banned over the years. Many appetite-suppressant medications that tamper with the body's serotonin levels have been withdrawn by the FDA, whereas those that alter levels of catecholamine are reported to have led to sleeplessness, nervousness and euphoria.

An extremely controversial appetite-suppressant, withdrawn from the market in the 1990s, was Fen-phen. This was a combination of two drugs - fenfluramine and phentermine.

A fatal lung disease called Primary Pulmonary Hypertension (PPH) was found to be associated with fenfluramine. Hence, not only was Fen-phen withdrawn from commercial sale by its manufacturers, but two other drugs, one that contained fenfluramine (Pondimin) and the other that contained dexfenfluramine (Redux), were withdrawn in 1997.

Drugs containing the appetite-suppressant phenylpropanolamine were banned in 2000 after they were found to precipitate hemorrhagic stroke. Similar concerns relating to ephedrine caused the FDA to ban this drug for use in dietary supplements in 2004.

But, it seems, the FDA has left a gaping loophole in its regulatory procedures for some prescription drugs, including diet pills. This allows their prescription for 'off-label' use. This basically means doctors can still prescribe them at will, a dangerous practice where doctors are allowed virtually free rein with these toxic chemical compounds.

No Miracle Cures

With a third of the American population obese and two-thirds overweight, this group of individuals is a happy hunting ground for doctors and drug manufacturers.

Some so-called weight-management plans that promise 'easy' weight loss recommend the use of antidepressants and amphetamines for weight-reduction. Antidepressants have been found to initially suppress appetite even though many overweight individuals tend to regain this lost weight while still taking these drugs.

Amphetamines, as mentioned earlier, have been banned for use as appetite-suppressants. But some doctors claiming to be weight-loss experts easily hand them out to desperate individuals looking for a 'miracle cure for obesity'.

Though there are no miracle cures, ironically, the search for anti-obesity drugs continues. Among these discoveries is the development of a nasal spray that is claimed to control eating and obesity.

The product (still being developed when this book was written) is reported to contain a protein hormone called PYY3–36.

The pharma company researching this drug claims that the product contains a naturally occurring hormone as opposed to synthetic hormones and other chemicals present in anti-obesity drugs on the market. If only losing weight was as easy as spraying protein into the nostrils!

Don't get me wrong. Science and research adds to our knowledge pool and we are constantly evolving in our understanding of the human body. But it is a moot point whether appetite-suppressants really work. Worse still, when men of science use their knowledge to profit, it usually means your health is at risk.

At the heart of the matter is the question: Should we tamper with the complex and delicate balance of hormones when there are natural ways to shed weight?

Doctors - much to the dismay of overweight individuals - have realized that after the initial loss of a few pounds with appetite suppressants, weight-loss seems to level off. Worse still, a lot of the weight shed also seems to come right back on!

Perhaps that is nature's way of saying that using these drugs is futile. Appetite-control or the hunger signal is a complex phenomenon and is driven by many hormones. You can't just turn off one hormone and expect to not feel hungry.

The body is driven towards eating as it needs nourishment. It seems like the failure to find a magic anti-obesity pill is but doomed to fail, as it rails against our very survival instinct.

Hunger Hormones

Appetite, satiety and metabolism are complex biochemical processes that cannot simply be turned on and turned off, as some would have the American population believe.

In this section, we will take a look at some of the body's natural hormones and the roles they play in regulating energy levels and triggering the hunger and satiety responses.

The biochemistry of appetite involves several hormones produced in different organs of the body. Hormones that play a direct role in metabolism and their impact on fat storage are: insulin, leptin and ghrelin.

Medical science has conclusively linked obesity to insulin-resistance (as in type 2 diabetes) and cardiovascular disease, which when present together are called the Metabolic Syndrome or, in medical slang, 'Diabesity'.

This is a modern disease caused mainly by two factors - a sedentary lifestyle and unhealthy Western diets high in refined carbohydrates and refined sugars and sweeteners such as high-fructose corn syrup.

Research has shown that the seeds of metabolic syndrome are sown early, where children are raised on a diet rich in refined carbohydrates and refined sugars. Some nutritionists would go so far as to say that more than saturated fats (unless these are also consumed in large quantities and regularly), it is refined carbohydrates and sugars that are the leading causes of metabolic syndrome.

In this section, we shall try and understand the link between insulin and obesity, the role insulin plays in regulating metabolism, and why the consumption of refined foods by overweight individuals is a self-defeating and lethal combination.

Insulin is a hormone and it is produced in the pancreas. It is the principal regulator of blood glucose or blood sugar levels.

When carbohydrates enter the small intestine, they are broken down into glucose. Glucose, in turn, is released into the bloodstream for transportation to the body's cells, which use it as fuel for energy.

Insulin basically makes glucose available to the cells, which are impermeable to the compound. Insulin binds to specific receptors in the cell membrane, thereby allowing the passage of glucose into the cell from the blood.

Individuals who are insulin-resistant are those whose cells do not respond to insulin. One reason is a significant reduction in the number of insulin-sensitive receptors in the cell membrane.

This has a cascading effect. Since the insulin doesn't work, blood sugar levels rise and the pancreas secretes more insulin, which ironically does not work either. This leads to abnormally high levels of insulin in the bloodstream and a vicious cycle and that is at the heart of type 2 diabetes.

But how does insulin-resistance promote weight gain? Without glucose, their basic fuel, the body's cells are starved of energy. They experience a famine and begin to crave for glucose. Hence, the body demands more food.

This stimulates the release of more insulin (which cannot be used). The excess glucose that builds up in the body is converted into fat. This fat is stored in the liver and adipose tissue. The result: obesity.

Hence, insulin-resistant individuals have high blood insulin levels, high blood glucose levels and excess fatty tissue.

Insulin-resistance also explains why overweight and obese individuals experience food cravings especially for carbohydrate-rich foods. Refined carbohydrates (processed foods) are a near-instant source of glucose. But as opposed to whole carbs, refined carbs (which most Americans are so addicted to) lead to another problem.

They cause blood sugar levels to surge suddenly, promoting a surge in insulin as well. To offset frequent insulin surges, the body's cells go into defensive mode and decrease the number of insulin receptors in their membranes. This worsens insulin-resistance.

Perhaps this explains the ironic cliché: 'The fatter you are, the fatter you get'.

Metabolic syndrome is characterized by the following:
- Excess abdominal fat or central adiposity
- High blood sugar
- High triglyceride levels
- Low HDL and high LDL
- High blood pressure

Metabolic syndrome is estimated to afflict 20–25percent of the American population.

Stress Can Make You Fat

Chronic stress and anxiety tend to pile on the pounds, a connection research studies have repeatedly demonstrated.

Emotional stress is a fact of modern life and it is something we all experience. Uncompromising demands at work, troubled family relationships, tangled personal relationships, and financial difficulties are only some of the sources of long-term anxiety that burden out minds and harm our health.

Temperament too plays an important role in how stressed we are. Some people are able to deal with stress better than others, while still others are chronic worry warts.

The relationship between stress and obesity is complex and, no, not all anxiety-prone individuals are overweight. But stress is often correlated with obesity.

Perhaps this is because, in addition to temperament, overweight individuals encounter more stress than other individuals. Being overweight itself invites other health problems; then there is the socially stressful aspect to obesity, and negative perceptions of the self that cause chronic anxiety and depression.

In an evolutionary sense, the stress response is a 'flight or fight' response or a survival response, where a stimulus like the detection of a predator once caused certain biochemical changes in the body that prepared early man to deal with any eventuality.

The stress response triggers the release of a natural steroid called cortisol, which triggers the liver to immediately release glucose into the bloodstream. This emergency response makes additional fuel readily available to the body so that it is flooded with energy to grapple with the stressor.

When the blood is flooded with glucose, the pancreas receives a signal to release insulin, causing an insulin surge. Increased insulin helps the body's cells convert glucose into energy.

Notice that the body responds in the same way as it does to surges and spikes of glucose and insulin when it is regularly fed refined carbohydrates and sugars (as described above). Over time, this leads to insulin-resistance, which once again, sets off the vicious cycle of hunger and obesity experienced in the metabolic syndrome.

Unlike our ancestors, we no longer encounter physical predators but the sources of emotional stress, fear and anxiety have multiplied manifold over time. Instead of cortisol surges, chronically anxious individuals have elevated levels of cortisol. This usually promotes insulin-resistance.

Stress also elevates levels of cholesterol, which in time leads to a condition called atherosclerosis or blocked arteries that cause hypertension and reduced blood supply to the heart.

Individuals who are overweight are often hit with a double-whammy. They tend to 'feed off stress' and rely on comfort food to make them feel better. Comfort food - potato chips, pasta, tortillas, baked food and colas - is rich in refined carbohydrates and sweeteners like high-fructose corn syrup.

These foods directly promote fatty build-up, fuelling adipose tissue, carbohydrate cravings and the vicious metabolic syndrome cycle.

All of a sudden, you find that you have fallen into a 'fat trap' and don't know how to get out. Under the circumstances, you are extremely vulnerable to the promotional spiel of weight-reduction programs and websites offering 'easy weight-loss tips'.

Alas, few desperate individuals realize it but they are simply feeding off the frenzy whipped up by clever marketing. Notice how none of these slimming programs mention health issues and how they readily dole out low-fat, low-carb and fat-burning 'formulae' that promise to whip you back into shape. Ouch!

Appetite: The Master Key

We have discussed the role of insulin in metabolism, blood glucose levels and insulin-resistance in obesity and metabolic disease. But it is the hypothalamus that keeps track of the body's nutritional needs, and the levels of different hormones, blood glucose and fatty acids.

This relatively small structure in the brain, which incidentally also regulates temperature, is the central processor or master controller that drives appetite and responds to satiety signals through complex biochemical pathways.

The pancreas and other organs directly involved in energy intake and metabolism merely do its bidding. This process of regulating energy balance is called homeostasis.

The hypothalamus is sensitive to two hormones in particular - leptin and ghrelin. Both these hormones are also sensitive to sleep patterns, which also influence eating habits.

The subjective feeling of hunger is your hypothalamus actually sensing that blood glucose levels have fallen. The liver, which converts food into glucose, then signals the lateral hypothalamus to prompt you either to open the refrigerator, serve yourself a meal or visit a fast-food restaurant.

The hormone leptin, manufactured in your body's fat cells, also plays a role in appetite. Low leptin levels signal the hypothalamus that the body needs more glucose.

After you eat, you begin to digest your meal and blood glucose levels rise. That is when the satiety response is triggered in the hypothalamus, and it signals you to stop eating.

This happens when the stomach and pancreas release a hormone called ghrelin, which acts on the ventromedial hypothalamus. When you are 'full', leptin is also released from the fat cells, signaling satiety.

Leptin and ghrelin act in opposing ways and when the level of one of these two hormones is low, the level of the other is elevated. Also, while ghrelin plays a greater role in stimulating appetite, leptin is believed to play a role in the satiety response.

Some studies suggest that overweight individuals who are insulin-resistant may also be leptin-resistant. When this is the case, the hypothalamus fails to recognize the satiety response generated by raised leptin levels. That is why overweight individuals continue eating. Their bodies cannot tell when they have eaten enough!

What does all this mean? The human body is naturally geared towards achieving a sense of balance or equilibrium. However, the hormones, neurotransmitters, organs and tissues in overweight individuals are functioning in ways that are not normal, thus causing your body to seek a skewed equilibrium.

When obesity is due to a malfunction in the hypothalamus-leptin-ghrelin pathway, the condition is referred to as 'hypothalamic obesity'.

This imbalance can be corrected by natural means that cleanse and detoxify the body. This, coupled with good nutrition and healthy levels of physical activity, restores your body to its natural and healthy way of functioning and optimal body weight.

Another gland that plays a crucial role in the body's metabolism is the thyroid. It is the largest gland in the body and is situated in the neck.

This gland is connected to weight loss or weight gain due to its role in regulating metabolism. It influences and controls other hormones in the body which determine the speed at which your body burns calories and uses energy.

When the thyroid malfunctions - due to either underproduction or overproduction of the hormone thyroxine - it results in either hypothyroidism or hyperthyroidism.

Individuals suffering from hypothyroidism have significantly low levels of thyroxin and metabolism. Cells grow sluggish, the brain slows down, muscle weakness sets in, and there is a general feeling of listlessness, fatigue and sometimes depression.

Hypothyroidism produces other symptoms as well such as intolerance to cold, constipation, falling hair, and dry skin.

These symptoms are the result of a lowered basal metabolic rate. This is the rate at which the body burns energy when inactive. So why does hypothyroidism lead to weight gain?

Since the body's cells grow sluggish and use less energy, there is extra fuel available in the body. Logically, you need to then eat less so that you don't generate too much fuel, right? Better still, you can exercise and burn the extra fuel.

The problem is that individuals who are overweight have other systems out of sync. They have long since lost the ability to burn excess fuel due to factors such as insulin resistance, leptin resistance, a fatty liver, or due to an overdependence on sweetened beverages and processed food.

With other metabolic processes already out of gear, the food consumed, and the energy thus generated, is too much for a body with an underactive thyroid gland. The excess fuel is therefore stored as fat.

Hypothyroidism has varied causes including adrenal fatigue, underproduction of thyroxin, exposure to certain metals such as mercury, stress, and nutritional imbalances which include deficiencies in iodine, zinc and Vitamins B, C and E, and excess soy consumption.

Apart from making sure you get enough of the vitamins and minerals your body needs, you might also want to eat some radish, eat sea vegetables which are high in iodine, occasionally eat some gelatine, and eliminate saturated fats and make sure you get enough coconut oil instead.

Obesity: Table Dressing

Another factor influencing obesity is humble table salt. Several studies have linked sodium intake to being overweight. I am reproducing the intriguing findings of a Finnish study done by two researchers of the University of Helsinki and the University of Kuopio, who published their findings in the journal *Progress in Cardiovascular Diseases* in 2006.

These researchers claim that a 30–35 percent reduction in salt intake in Finland over a 30-year period led to a dramatic 75–80 percent decrease in the incidence of stroke and coronary disease across the population.

The study goes on to quote the American Salt Institute, a non-profit organization, to say that the salt intake in the US doubled between the mid-'80s and late '90s. This coincides perfectly with the dramatic jump in obesity figures for both men and women in the US.

The Finnish researchers have an interesting interpretation for their findings. They point out that increased salt intake leads to increased thirst. And to satiate their thirst, the average American almost instinctively reaches out for a cola or another type of artificially sweetened beverage.

Where does the excess salt come from? A large percentage of the average American's salt intake comes from processed foods, 20 percent from meat and meat products, and about 35 percent from breakfast cereals.

The study does not claim to conclusively link salt to processed foods and obesity. But the conclusions are nonetheless provocative.

Also, it is a scientific fact that salt makes an individual thirsty. When salt levels are elevated, they signal a state of dehydration and the body tries to hold on to as much water as possible to neutralize the sodium.

Not doing so would raise the body's acidic levels dangerously and upset the pH (acid-alkaline) balance which needs to be maintained within a very narrow range. To reduce fluid output, the blood vessels constrict and this, in turn, leads to hypertension.

Both fluid retention and hypertension are closely related to obesity. In fact, some researchers claim that as much as 75 percent of individuals who are detected with hypertension are overweight.

Chapter 6: Surgery: Fatal Fix?

Stitched & Stapled

There are only two reasons I can think of that account for the huge success of weight-loss surgery in the United States - the Western world's obsession with quick-fix solutions due to an unwillingness to adopt an approach that requires an iota of effort, and the mind-boggling profits that surgeons make promoting this barbaric practice.

Yet here are the cold, hard facts:

Mortality Rate: Roughly 1-3 percent of individuals undergoing weight-loss surgery die within a few years after the procedure.

Additional Surgery: As many as 22 percent patients suffer complications post-surgery while still in hospital; 40 percent report complications within the first six months of surgery; and 20 percent need additional follow-up surgery to fix the complications due to the surgery.

'Too Successful': 30 percent of patients develop nutritional deficiencies such as anemia and osteoporosis. Sometimes, the surgery is so 'successful' that patients suffer, and even perish from, severe malnutrition

Failure Rate: If you don't die of it or fall seriously ill, you are likely to be back where you started. That is because 25 percent of individuals who undergo weight-reduction procedures do not lose the weight they expected to shed. This could either be because the surgery itself was unsuccessful or the patient failed to maintain the prescribed diet post-surgery.

'Bariatric surgery' is a term used to describe several procedures that surgically remove large sections of the digestive tract to essentially reduce the intake of food.

It works on two simple, if savage, principles: forcibly reduce appetite and food intake to drastically cut down on the calories you ingest, and restrict the ability of the now-brutalized digestive tract to absorb nutrients from food.

For many morbidly obese individuals, surgery is the last resort, after numerous attempts at dieting, exercising and pharmaceutical drugs fail to work. Desperate to lead normal lives, patients consent to going under the knife, allowing a doctor to reach into their abdomen and rip out vital organs, and twist, turn, staple and stitch together what is left inside into an unnatural mess.

In other words, some obese individuals - at least 200,000 a year in the US - are making a conscious choice to be severely crippled and maimed. If these sound like harsh words, I am not exaggerating.

Being morbidly obese can be life-threatening and there is a host of health issues associated with the condition. This apart from the socially and personally challenging nature of the disease. But before we discuss alternative ways to approach this issue, let us take a brief look at why weight-reduction surgery appears to work.

There are numerous variations that go by different names such as gastric bypass surgery, biliopancreatic diversion, duodenal switch, stomach stapling, vertical banded gastroplasty and sleeve gastrectomy.

Another option, still being tested in Europe, is the 'gastric pacer', which is implanted on the surface of the stomach, in much the same way as a pacemaker is implanted in the heart.

This gadget connects with your nervous system and connects to the brain to mimic the feeling of satiety. On other words, it makes you feel full even when you are not eating.

Contrast this with the complicated process of energy homeostasis that doctors are still unable to fully understand. As discussed later in Chapter 11, the processes of energy regulation are dominated by two hormones, ghrelin and leptin, which work through a complicated series of pathways controlled by the hypothalamus.

Despite decades of research, scientists are yet to uncover the exact mechanisms by which these hormones work, the neurotransmitters involved and neural pathways that relay the messages of satiety and hunger.

Several pharmaceutical drugs have also tried to tinker with this delicate balance and have failed. Now here's an electrical gadget that purports to alter a process that nature is yet to reveal to medical science!

Strip away the fancy medical jargon of weight-loss surgery and what you are left with is a stomach that is reduced to around 15 percent of its original size, a small intestine (the seat of digestion and immunity) that has had essential segments like the duodenum removed.

Not only is your food intake drastically reduced, but what is left of your digestive tract is also unable to effectively process, metabolize and absorb what does go into it. Weight-loss surgery therefore radically alters your body's biochemistry and metabolism in a way that nature never intended.

Not surprisingly, nature will revolt. Though bariatric surgery is reported to bring about dramatic results - a reduction by as much as half or more of body weight - it is also associated with dangerous medical complications.

Remember, weight-loss surgery is irreversible. You simply cannot re-attach a part of the small intestine that has been so nonchalantly snipped off or expect a portion of your stomach, rendered redundant for several months, to start working again.

Return to Barbarism

One of the most common life-threatening consequences of gastric bypass surgery is malnutrition. While a part of your post-op diet is bound to include vitamin and mineral supplements - a brutalized digestive tract can no longer absorb these elements from the little food that you now eat - it is not really all that simple.

The human body is not a machine that responds to simple addition, subtraction and a pinch of minerals. The National Institute of Diabetes and Digestive and Kidney Diseases admits that 30 percent patients who undergo bariatric surgery could suffer serious nutritional deficiency disorders, including anemia and osteoporosis, and an intolerance to red meat, milk products, and other food types.

Another common side-effect of weight-reduction surgery is hypoglycemia or low blood sugar. Symptoms of hypoglycemia include confusion, lightheadedness, rapid heart rate, the shakes, sweating and excessive hunger. If not treated immediately, patients could slip into a coma as do diabetic individuals whose blood glucose tends to fall to dangerously low levels.

At face value, it is logical to assume that if your food intake is drastically reduced, your blood sugar levels will fall. But it is much more complicated than that. Research at the Mayo Clinic discovered a link between hypoglycemia and a condition called hyperinsulinemia, a potentially life-threatening combination of diseases.

Hyperinsulinemia is a condition where there is too much insulin circulating in the bloodstream. Insulin is a hormone that helps the body's cells absorb glucose through the cell membrane.

Post-surgery, the quantum of insulin now released by the pancreas is too much proportionate to the too-little glucose now produced by reduced food intake. The body simply does not have sufficient glucose that needs to be absorbed.

The second reason for abnormally high insulin levels post-surgery is that obese individuals tend to grow more insulin-producing islet cells in the pancreas. This is an abnormal adjustment the body makes when food intake is consistently elevated. Post-surgery, despite the dramatic reduction in food intake, the pancreas continues to produce elevated levels of insulin.

The Mayo Clinic research also found that gastric bypass surgery could actually stimulate the islet cells to proliferate or lead to these cells turning overactive. This, in turn, causes dangerous levels of insulin to circulate in the blood.

The abnormal growth of pancreatic cells is called nesidioblastosis. The only solution to this is to remove the pancreas, which apart from producing insulin, also manufactures many digestive enzymes.

Now here is a comment on how little we know about the consequences of altering the internal architecture of the human body. Though gastric bypass surgery has been around for five decades, the link between hyperinsulinemia and hypoglycemia in gastric bypass patients was discovered as recently as 2005.

Weight-loss surgery results in several other serious side-effects. One of these is called 'gastric dumping', whose symptoms include lightheadedness, abdominal cramping, vomiting, diarrhea and reflux.

Gastric dumping occurs because an abnormally reduced digestive tract forces a severely shrunken stomach to dump undigested food into a shortened small intestine, clogging it and leading to congestion.

Food is therefore not metabolized properly. Undigested food, whose nutrients cannot be absorbed through the walls of the small intestine, tends to back up, leading to gastric reflux or the backing up of food into the shrunken stomach.

It doesn't end there. Other serious complications that arise from surgically joining the stomach and the intestine include hernias, pneumonia, infections, abdominal abscesses, bowel obstruction, stomach ulcers, abdominal bleeding and gallstones.

Gastrointestinal leaks are a major consequence of bariatric surgery. Leaks could occur at any portion that has been surgically cut and re-attached to another portion of the digestive system.

A leak suggests that the connection between any two parts is either splitting or tearing at the seams or that these two parts have not been effectively stitched or stapled together.

Also remember, since most of the small intestine has been removed, the bowels are now too close to the stomach, and this may cause waste from the bowels to back up into the abdominal area.

The undigested, rotting waste invariably leads to infection or even sepsis that could prove fatal if not detected and treated in time. The only remedy for this is emergency surgery.

Of Profits & Fraudsters

Despite the overwhelming evidence that it will probably cause severe medical complications, more and more morbidly obese individuals are opting for this life-threatening remedy in the hope that they can lead a normal, healthy life.

And why not? After all, doctors, hospitals and clinics and even insurance companies are earning millions of dollars from these and other unnecessary surgical procedures.

Topping the list of needless surgeries in the US is coronary bypass for men and hysterectomies and C-Sections for women. Set this against the backdrop of a population that is growing increasingly unhealthy and the fears associated with health, and the medical fraternity has a fertile hunting ground to play predator.

Add to this the aggressive marketing of these surgeries and you've got a desperate section of the population, many gullible and ill-informed, who are willing to shell out an average $30,000 to get their internal organs badly messed up. And that amount is minus post-op treatment and possible 'remedial' surgeries.

Internet advertising and private clinics use publicity material that liberally uses Hollywood actors as 'model patients' of weight-loss surgery, thus turning a barbaric practice into something that sounds even desirable.

When slick marketing comes from advertising professionals and the Internet, you don't really expect them to substantiate their claims. But when outrageous statements are made by a medical journal, it is a symptom of the sickness that has taken root in the medical fraternity. Read on.

The January 2009 issue of *Pediatrics*, the journal of the American Academy of Pediatrics, carried a report titled 'Reversal of Type 2 Diabetes Mellitus and Improvements in Cardiovascular Risk Factors After Surgical Weight Loss in Adolescents'.

The claim that weight-loss surgery could actually 'reverse type 2 diabetes' pertained to a study conducted at the Cincinnati Children's Hospital Medical Center, one of five medical centers awarded a $3.9-million grant by the National Institutes of Health, an agency of the US Department of Health.

The study, which received its funding in 2006, is expected to be completed in 2011. Yet, three years before that deadline, in a media release dated December 29, 2008, Cincinnati Children's made these astonishing claims: that the study it was conducting noted a 'dramatic, often immediate remission' of type 2 diabetes in the - hold your breath - 11 adolescents who had undergone the surgery as part of the study.

The Cincinnati Children's added: "The results have been quite dramatic, and to our knowledge, there are no other anti-diabetic therapies that result in more effective and long-term control than that seen with bariatric surgery."

Calling its study a "breakthrough", the release said that "remaining diabetes-free is well worth" having the surgery.

Despite the weight of evidence that bariatric surgery can cause hypoglycemia and other serious medical complications, the Surgical Director of the Surgical Weight Loss Program for Teens, Cincinnati Children's, was quoted as saying: "In addition to the impressive weight loss and type 2 diabetes results, patients undergoing the gastric bypass surgery also showed significant improvement in blood pressure, insulin, glucose, cholesterol and triglyceride levels."

The media release had set up readers for these mind-boggling claims by first stating an established medical fact -

that the rise in type 2 diabetes in obese American children and teenagers was a worrying and growing problem. Having struck the right emotional cord, it hoped to gain credibility for claims that the rest of medical science is yet to establish.

When men in white coats offer weight-loss surgery as the answer to two alarming health issues among a vulnerable section of the population, gullible parents are liable to bite the bait. Needless to say, some of their children pay with their lives for trusting so readily.

Weight-reduction surgery is still not a procedure of choice among adolescents though in absolute terms, it is estimated that about 2,700 teenagers undergo these procedures every year. But with fantastic claims being made by medical centers such as Cincinnati Children's and other medical facilities, it could become a more popular option among youngsters as well.

Here is another equally ludicrous claim made by another study, this one conducted at Monash University in Melbourne, Australia. Published in January 2008, in the *Journal of the American Medical Association*, the study claims that patients who underwent gastric banding (a type of bariatric surgery) "were five times more likely to have their diabetes go into long-term remission than those who engaged in conventional weight-loss therapies".

Calling it a "world-first study", researchers studied 60 patients over two years and found that 73 percent of them had "gone into long-term" remission for type 2 diabetes compared to only 13 percent who underwent conventional therapy.

Apart from the hollow claims made by the study, the most incriminating fact is that Dr John Dixon, the lead author of the study and an obesity researcher at Monash University, had received research grants and speaker's fees from the company that makes the gastric bands, Allergan Health.

Dr Dixon was therefore obliged to make these claims, and was clearly happy to do so. After all, he was quoted in the media as saying, "I think diabetes surgery will become common within the next few years."

Moreover, the doctors who wrote the editorial in the *Journal*, said of the study: "The insights already beginning to be gained by studying surgical interventions for diabetes may be the most profound since the discovery of insulin."

These same doctors, or editorial writers, also admitted to having accepted travel grants from Allergan and other companies to attend a conference on diabetes surgery in Rome.

There are three reasons why I have mentioned these two studies in such detail. Both studies were conducted by reputed medical institutions and published in respected medical journals. Yet both the institutions and journals have been extremely irresponsible - if not downright unethical - in making these claims.

The second reason is to illustrate how deceptive the 'gospel truth' can be. When you read claims as seemingly profound as these, you simply must be discerning. Ask yourself whether there could be a hidden motive. Ask yourself who might stand to gain. Ask yourself if you have been given all the facts. And always conduct your own research before you blindly accept what you read - even in the hallowed *Journal of the American Medical Association*!

The third point I want to make is that there is no such thing as 'remission' in diabetes. Also, gastric banding is *not* more effective than natural methods to control and keep type 2 diabetes in check. In fact, it is a barbaric procedure that should not be conducted on the human body.

However, by using words such as 'remissions', a term conventional medicine usually associates with cancer, the researchers hoped to evoke a strong emotional response to make their statements sound more credible.

Here is another surprising proponent of weight-loss surgery - the American public health insurance system. In 2006, the Centers for Medicare and Medicaid Services (CMS), which determines policy for the US federal health program, announced new measures to expand its coverage to bariatric surgery under health insurance schemes. Till then, public health insurance did not recognize these ruthless surgeries as being essential healthcare procedures.

But by 2006, the number of obese individuals going under the knife for weight loss, and paying for it themselves, had (not coincidentally) leapfrogged. What better way to earn huge profits than to cover it under the public health care system?

According to the new rules, public health insurers were now willing to cover individuals for bariatric surgery if they underwent the procedures in "high-volume centers from highly qualified surgeons (as certified by the American College of Surgeons or the American Society for Bariatric Surgery)".

Beneficiaries were to have a Body Mass Index or BMI of 35 or higher, and to have exhibited a serious health condition in addition to morbid obesity such as hypertension, coronary artery disease or osteoarthritis.

Only three types of surgeries would be covered: Roux-en-Y gastric bypass, gastric banding and biliopancreatic diversion with a duodenal switch. Of course, these covered the most popular procedures.

Then, in February 2009, CMS amended its criteria and announced that it would not cover weight-reduction surgery "when it is used to treat type 2 diabetes in a beneficiary with a BMI below 35".

With further data coming in on these procedures and with further market research, expect the rules to be further refined. CMS has its eye, not on your health, but firmly on profits. And how exactly does it do that?

As with all other medical procedures covered by health insurance, insurers offer medical cover and then devise tiny legal fine print to deny the thousands of claims pouring in.

This is not a new gimmick. The US public health insurance system is designed to sabotage insurance claims to carefully nurture the illusion that it is concerned about your health while laughing all the way to the bank.

'Craving' Morbidity

Perhaps another reason bariatric surgery is so tempting is that it is marketed as an instant and permanent solution to obesity. In a society where so much can be achieved at the touch of a button or the click of the mouse, few seem inclined to invest time or energy in achieving their goals, and that includes health.

But the solutions need not be drastic; neither do they require a sudden burst of energy to implement. When you think about what made you morbidly obese in the first place, the finger for most individuals points to an overdependence on processed foods and beverages, and physical inactivity.

Processed foods like sugary breakfast cereals, pastas, pies, pizzas and nachos, chocolate chip cookies, crisps, fries and salted potato chips, and sandwich and burger buns are all made of refined carbohydrates and starch.

The key to understanding obesity - and reversing it - lies in food cravings and their effects on metabolism. Food cravings are caused by a variety of factors and it is important to identify what type of craving you experience and the biochemical process that powers it.

The most common type of craving is for carbohydrates and sugar which send insulin levels out of gear. Refined carbs, refined sugar, sweeteners in colas and sodas, consumed compulsively and consistently over a period of time cause changes in your brain, blood and body chemistry. This, in turn, leads to food cravings and compulsive eating.

When the level of toxicity is almost more than your body can handle, anything you eat is interpreted as a potential threat or poison, leading your body to pad up with more adipose to protect itself.

After a while, it may not take too many carbs or too much sugar to put on weight. That is because you are already caught in an unhealthy carb/sugar-insulin loop.

This is how it works. Too much refined carbohydrates and refined sugar drives up insulin levels, so that when carbs and sugar are converted into glucose, which is transported to the body's cell through the bloodstream, insulin helps the cells absorb it for use as energy.

When you over-consume refined carbohydrates and sugar, insulin levels rise dramatically. This causes an 'energy rush'. Suddenly elevated levels of insulin then cause the cells to absorb blood glucose quickly, leading to a 'crash'. The resultant fatigue, tiredness, lethargy and hunger lead your body to crave more carbs and sugar to raise blood sugar levels.

But by sheer force of habit, your pancreas begins to anticipate a sudden overload of carbs every single time, and it releases a rush of insulin, even if you eat only a little. Elevated insulin levels drive up appetite and hence, you eat more, and more. And the vicious cycle of energy spikes and crashes continues in a failed attempt to balance blood sugar and insulin levels.

In the meantime, what happens to the excess glucose in the bloodstream? It is stored in the fat tissue or adipose.

Over time, the body's cells, to protect themselves from a glucose overload, also reduce the number of glucose receptors on their external membranes. You then develop insulin resistance and you are also on the road to developing metabolic syndrome.

Now your insulin, blood glucose, several endocrine functions and neurotransmitters are thrown out of gear. The only shock absorber, so to speak, against this assault is your adipose tissue, which keeps building to keep protecting. Hence, overweight turns to obesity and obesity morphs into morbid obesity.

Don't forget, this is simultaneously fuelling more and more internal congestion and a consequent build-up of toxins. When the toxicity crisis spills over, you fall seriously sick.

Carbohydrate cravings also result from low levels of a neurotransmitter in the brain called serotonin. This neurotransmitter serves many functions, including regulation of mood and sleep. When levels of serotonin dip, you feel moody, depressed and irritable. When serotonin levels are elevated, you experience a sense of well-being, calm and relaxation.

Women with Seasonal Affective Disorder (SAD) experience feelings of depression caused by lowered levels of serotonin. It is called 'seasonal' because this disorder usually manifests itself during the winter months when sunlight is weak.

This is no coincidence. Sunlight stimulates the production of serotonin and is therefore a natural 'upper'! There is another way to increase the levels of this neurotransmitter in the brain - by eating carbohydrates.

Hence, your carb craving might just be fuelled by low serotonin levels. Serotonin is naturally synthesized by the brain from an essential amino acid called tryptophan. The body receives this amino acid from the proteins you eat. But since tryptophan is also used for other purposes such as to make other proteins or Vitamin B3, it is not always available to the brain in sufficient quantities to synthesize serotonin.

So why doesn't the body instead crave protein, a natural source of tryptophan, and why does it demand carbohydrates? This happens because tryptophan is very sensitive to the blood-brain barrier, or the brain's natural filter. It is always competing with other amino acids to get past the blood-brain barrier. Hence, eating more proteins means also ingesting various types of competing amino acids. Tryptophan usually loses out.

Alternatively, eating carbohydrates results in elevated levels of insulin, which clears away the competing amino acids and allows tryptophan to penetrate the blood-brain barrier.

Chocolate cravings work in much the same way, allowing the required quantity of tryptophan to make it to the brain to produce serotonin. Chocolate also contains caffeine, which is addictive as well. This explains why many depressed individuals are compulsive chocolate eaters. It makes them feel better.

Sounds complicated? This only demonstrates how sensitive the human body is to the food we eat. Despite these complexities and the supreme dexterity with which it simultaneously balances thousands of chemical processes, we abuse it with processed foods and beverages, highly acidic foods and irregular eating and sleeping habits.

What you do not realize every time you take a bite of pizza or pie is that with every slice or morsel, you are throwing your body's biochemistry into disarray. We do not realize this because we do not experience the effects of a disturbed metabolism or biochemistry immediately and directly.

And when the toxicity crisis crosses your body's threshold and results in the self-defeating obesity cycle, many opt for the barbaric practice of weight-loss surgery!

Why Not Nature?

I fail to understand why anyone would choose to allow a doctor to cut out and mash up their internal organs, further mess up their biochemistry and claim to have solved their obesity problem, while leaving them open to further chemical imbalances, infection, and even possible death.

Rule number one: cut out processed foods and sugary beverages from your diet immediately, and replace them with healthy choices such as fruits and vegetables. Eliminating refined carbohydrates and sugar, high-fructose corn syrup and artificial additives, not to mention greasy animal proteins and fats, from your diet will bring about profound and immediate changes in your body.

It will kill food cravings and also kick start the process of weight loss. This also needs to be accompanied by other natural remedies which I have explained later in this book.

Along with a change in diet, it is important to stabilize appetite and blood glucose levels by eating small portions of nutritious foods throughout the day. Individuals who suffer from nutritional deficiencies or gross imbalances in certain chemicals may require nutritional supplements until these imbalances are also restored.

Natural supplements, once identified, are available in stores and must be taken only as per your body's requirements.

Carbohydrate cravings can also be eliminated by engaging in regular physical activity or exercise (Chapter 12: Energize, Not Exercise). Even an easy stroll daily can profoundly alter brain chemistry and stimulate the production of healthful brain chemicals. This is so rewarding that you will spontaneously feel encouraged to make healthier dietary and other lifestyle choices.

But most doctors will not offer you these choices. Apart from trotting out the usual 'spiel' about diet and exercise in five minutes flat, they usually go on to advise morbidly obese individuals to opt for surgery as a 'last resort'.

Violating ethical guidelines, many surgeons do not explain the risks and consequences of such radical surgery to patients, afraid that this might scare them off.

Modern medical practitioners pushing bariatric surgery are profit-driven, faced as they are with another threat. This comes from 'medical tourism', a growing industry where hi-tech (and not-so-hi-tech) medical procedures are outsourced to countries where they cost significantly less.

Many Asian countries perform bariatric and other surgeries at a fraction of what it costs in the US. These countries, like India, Singapore and the Philippines, have doctors trained in Western medicine and are equipped with state-of-the-art medical facilities comparable in some centers to those in the West.

Encouraging this trend, some private insurers in the US have begun to offer medical cover for certain medical procedures, such as coronary bypass, if they are performed outside the country. Corporate firms are also jumping onto the 'medical tourism' bandwagon, encouraging their staff to opt for such schemes.

It became common practice many years ago for Westerners opting for cosmetic surgery to head East, thanks to the cost benefits and medical expertise available in some Asian countries. Now knee- and hip-replacement surgery, dental procedures, organ transplants, wellness treatments, and, of course, weight-loss surgeries are routinely outsourced.

I can never understand the justification offered by individuals who opt for weight-reduction surgery, that they 'have tried everything'. I can say with certainty that these individuals have not give nature a fair chance.

Sometimes the solutions are so simple and freely available that we often fail to see them. As discussed earlier in this book, overweight and obese individuals are suffering from a toxicity crisis, turning adipose tissue into a system that stores poisons so that they do not enter the bloodstream.

Apart from an unhealthy diet, other reasons for a toxic build-up include bad sleeping habits, overstimulating the senses, chronic stress and emotional toxicity.

Since a toxic lifestyle by definition implies that it has developed over the years, reversing this process by natural means could take a few weeks or months.

It all boils down to a matter of choice. But many overweight and obese individuals may not make the natural, healthy choice simply because they do not have access to information about foods, healing, weight loss and nutrition.

They therefore do not realize that there is a perfectly natural way to return to a natural and healthy life without bariatric surgery.

Let me put it this way. Starving to death does not constitute a healthy or natural weight loss plan. The human body does not have excess stomach or intestinal tissue. No one is born with excess stomach tissue to allow more than three-quarters of this organ to be removed.

Reversing obesity is a nutritional and behavioral challenge. It cannot be 'fixed' by removing vital organs from the body.

Chapter 7: Stuck on Sugar?

Sucrose Shock

It's a sugar-coated myth that the Western world has been sold on ever since the advent of television - that sugar is an instant and good source of energy. Well, that is true, except for one little word disguised so cleverly by those snowy white grains - refined.

It is a word that spells trouble, big trouble. And its effects on the palate are so powerful that refined sugar became one of the key ingredients in America's obesity epidemic.

In the course of this discussion on sugar, we shall look at the myth that sugar is a natural ingredient. We shall also examine recent findings which reveal that refined white sugar is more damaging to the body than researchers have thus far suspected.

Later in this chapter, we shall also discuss another sweetener - high-fructose corn sugar - why it was such a 'find' for America, and why a 'subsidy' is sometimes no less than a 'bribe'.

Refined white sugar is commonly used as an ingredient in foods as well as a table condiment. That is what most people assume, at least. But the fact is that refined sugar is liberally used also in bread, breakfast cereal, mayonnaise, salad dressing, peanut butter, ketchup, spaghetti sauce, microwave meals and a host of other processed food products.

But just why is refined sugar so damaging to our health? There are various types of sugars - glucose (found in grains, fruits and plants; natural blood sugar; (also synthetically produced), fructose (fruit sugar), lactose (milk sugar), maltose (malt sugar) and dextrose (corn sugar made synthetically from starch).

Sucrose occurs naturally in many green plants including different types of palms, the sugar maple, and beet and cane. Cane and beet are the commercially significant sources.

However, when the word 'sucrose' occurs on food labels, it usually refers to a factory-made product that treats cane juice with sulphur dioxide, phosphoric acid and calcium hydroxide, chemicals the body could well do without.

That's because refined white sugar dumps 'empty' calories into the body. These are also called 'naked' calories because the refining process strips the cane juice of all its nutritional content - vitamins, minerals, salts, fiber and proteins.

So when you eat or drink anything with refined sugar, you are literally dumping in calories without any nutrients. Sure, the food, tea and cakes taste sumptuous but think about how they are ruining your health.

Make no mistake. Stripped and devoid of its life force, those tiny white cubes and crystals are literally shocking your body into taking certain emergency measures to protect itself. With every successive teaspoon of refined sugar, you are also taking a step closer to type 2 diabetes, obesity or heart disease.

When you ingest any food or beverage with refined sugar used as a sweetener, the sugar hit your body receives creates an immediate chemical imbalance. This is because, unlike foods and vegetables, refined sugar is devoid of vitamins and minerals.

Refined sugar, due to its chemical composition, also makes the blood acidic and alters its acid-alkaline balance. Since this balance is critical and delicately maintained, the body almost instantly begins to draw on its reserves of sodium, potassium and magnesium, calcium (from your bones and teeth) and B complex vitamins from the nervous system to return the blood to the required acid-alkaline equilibrium.

When consumed in large doses and consistently in the form of processed foods, candy and cookies and colas, your body is getting an overdose of refined sugar. The body begins to dump the excess sugar in the liver in the form of glycogen.

When the liver is saturated, this organ releases the extra glycogen into the bloodstream in the form of fatty acids, which are stored in the abdomen, buttocks, breasts and thighs as adipose tissue or fat cells.

Make cola and cookies part of your daily diet and the fatty acids are diverted to organs such as the heart and kidneys. These organs get congested and accumulate fatty tissue in and around them. Next, they begin to degenerate.

Eventually, the circulatory and lymphatic systems get overloaded and the toxicity crisis spills over until finally, something gives way.

The sugar hit provided by refined sugar (just like refined carbohydrates) produces a sudden and sharp increase in blood sugar. This leads to a sudden and sharp release of insulin from the pancreas to transport the sudden surge of glucose in the blood to the body's cells. As a result, there is a sudden drop in blood sugar, which the body experiences as a 'food famine'.

These surges and crashes, coupled with the lack of micro-nutrients in the blood, lead to food cravings. Note, cravings do not result from the absence of nutrition (that is malnutrition); they are caused by an imbalance in nutrients being ingested. It is the body's way of demanding what you are depriving it of.

The irony is that your body demands more sugar (or carbohydrates). But instead of the organic and whole form of sugar and carbohydrates it requires, you feed it with even more refined sugar (and refined carbs), creating a loop of deprivation leading to more deprivation.

If this see-saw effect continues over several years, it permanently disrupts the insulin-blood glucose balance. This eventually leads to your body becoming resistant to insulin. So now, you are not just overweight but likely to turn diabetic too. Insulin resistance is at the heart of type 2 diabetes.

In some individuals, overconsumption of refined sugar over the years could also lead to hypogylcemia. Yes, sugar can lead to a serious sugar deficit (in the blood)! This happens because when there is a sugar hit, increased insulin sweeps away glucose from the bloodstream so fast that it could lead to a dangerous drop in blood sugar.

The damage doesn't stop there. Refined sugar also interferes with the way cholesterol and fatty acids are metabolized, leading to elevated levels of serum triglycerides.

It leaves the body's immune system deficient and defeated. Why does this happen? When blood sugar levels rise beyond the healthy limit, glucose molecules compete with those of Vitamin C to enter the cells. That is because both glucose molecules and Vitamin C have a similar chemical structure. After a point, the glucose inevitably wins.

Since Vitamin C keeps white blood cells healthy, depriving the body of this vital vitamin weakens immunity and leaves you vulnerable to falling ill.

Vitamin C also facilitates fat metabolism and protects tissues from free radical damage. It strengthens the nervous system by converting certain amino acids into neurotransmitters. It also helps wounds to heal, combats inflammation and pain, and is required for healthy bones.

By eating too many cakes and cookies and then washing them down with a can of cola, you are actually setting yourself up for disease - any type of disease.

Now the more sugar you consume, the happier the sugar lobby. And World War I provided them with the perfect opportunity to drive the point home - that sugar was an instant source of energy. So we return to the myth we opened this chapter with.

Refined sugar provides an 'energy rush' within minutes. Contrast this with the gradual release of glucose due to the relatively slow process of digestion and metabolism of complex sugars and starches that are found in vegetables and whole grains.

Soldiers in the war were fed sugar to boost energy while in combat, thereby also boosting a half-truth that sugar is great fuel for stamina.

Unfortunately, we have come to regard the human body as a checking account. It is something that America of the 1920s is guilty of. It was then that the relationship between obesity and diabetes became apparent. And the culprit, doctors said, was calories.

So calorie counting became fashionable as did weight-loss products, weight-loss manuals and weight-loss 'experts'. Yes, counting calories became something of a national preoccupation.

It is a trend that continues today, much to the delight of food and beverage manufacturers who use the term 'calories' to disguise the rest of the poisonous ingredients with which they lace processed and packaged food. And an ill-informed public has been, quite literally, feeding off this drivel for more than four decades.

This trickery is best reflected in food labels (with the tacit approval of the Food and Drug Administration or FDA) that are deliberately designed to confuse.

Here is one ploy manufacturers routinely use to cloak the refined sugar content in foods. While labeling a product that contains both refined sugar and carbohydrates, they lump the sugar with the carbs. (Remember, carbohydrates such as potatoes, rice and wheat contain sugars and starch) Deliciously devious, isn't it?

The fact is that more than half the carbohydrates you consume in processed foods are in the form of factory-made sugars (sucrose, high-fructose corn syrup, etc) added as sweetening agents.

Also, did you know that the following common food products in your local supermarket contain refined sugar? Canned products such as fruits, vegetables and tomato juice, cereals, soups, certain types of meats, peanut butter, pizza, salad dressings, and spaghetti sauce. Why, even a spoon of ketchup contains a teaspoon of processed sugar. So does your spicy chili dog, which has quite a generous portion of this refined chemical.

If this is not downright diabolical, read on and discover some stunning facts about another favorite of the food-processing industry - high-fructose corn syrup.

Fructose: Corn Con

The 1970s were a watershed decade for the American food processing industry as well as the average American. It will always be flagged as the decade when Japanese scientists made a landmark discovery - how to artificially convert corn starch into a delicious sweetener that would also enhance food and beverage flavors and, with its preservative effect, also increase their shelf life.

The new discovery was called high-fructose corn syrup (HFCS), a sweetener that became Enemy Number One in America's battle with obesity.

But more than its chemical properties, it was the economics of HFCS that really made this sweetener click. It worked for food manufacturers, the American government and consumers.

Finally, here was a sweetener whose economics benefited everyone, something that could replace expensive cane sugar, which was then being used as the primary sweetener in processed foods and beverages.

Cane sugar is imported by the US and the high tariff was eating into the profits of the food manufacturing industry. Corn starch, on the other hand, was already being indigenously produced (corn is one of America's primary crops). HFCS means major cost savings for everyone!

What is HFCS?

Some basics first. Fructose, as a natural sugar, is abundantly present in fruit. It is what makes fruit taste sweet. But fruit also contains lots of plant fiber (among other natural nutrients), which regulates the release of this natural sweetener and energy source into the bloodstream.

The fructose in HFCS is not natural at all. In fact, it is nothing like the fructose that occurs in fruits. It is a synthetically produced molecule made by enzymes that convert the glucose in corn starch and corn syrup into something the processed foods industry calls 'fructose'.

The resultant syrup is 90 percent fructose, which is further processed with untreated syrup (containing only glucose) into a mixture that is 42 or 55 percent fructose. The rest is glucose.

Table sugar or refined white sugar has a similar composition, being made up of both glucose and fructose. The difference is that HFCS is present in almost every carbonated and fruity beverage that you drink (unless it contains the even-more damaging artificial sweetener called aspartame) and is perhaps even more addictive than refined white sugar.

Also, since HFCS is one of the main ingredients in sodas, you're actually drinking your calories - teaspoonfuls of them with each drink - rather than eating them slowly in food as nature intended.

Why HFCS is Sweet Trouble

The trouble with HFCS is that it is metabolized into fats and triglycerides more readily and rapidly than refined sugar. Also, because most fructose is consumed in liquid form - as fruit juice or soda - its harmful metabolic effects are magnified.

Unlike refined sugar, HFCS does not turn off appetite. It makes the body resistant to leptin, the 'satiety' hormone that regulates appetite.

So with every processed meal you eat - cakes and cookies, jellies, baked dishes, yoghurt and even bread and meats - your taste buds are enjoying something that is sumptuous but your stomach and small intestine are filling up with something that that is nutritionally empty, that promotes obesity, metabolic syndrome, diabetes, kidney disease, osteoarthritis and other diseases; *and* that is addictive because you never know when your body has eaten enough!

Recent studies indicate that HFCS could be much more damaging than was previously known. Two research studies, the results of which were announced in September 2009, have found a connection between HFCS and hypertension.

HFCS & Hypertension: Scientists from the University of Colorado-Denver conducted their research at the Mateo Orfila Hospital in Spain, where they studied 74 men who were administered 200 grams of fructose a day in addition to their regular diet. This was well above the 50–70 gm of fructose consumed by most American adults every day.

Presenting their findings before the American Heart Association in September, the researchers found that the group of men who received the additional fructose showed a significant increase in blood pressure, while those who did not consume the extra fructose displayed normal blood pressure levels.

Another group of researchers in Ohio studied the effects of fructose mixed with water administered to mice. Extending the results of their study to human beings, the researchers suggest that people who consume junk food and soda at night are more likely to gain weight than those who don't.

HFCS & Paralysis: Colas and processed foods that contain fructose could also lead to muscle fatigue and in some cases, even muscle paralysis. This was reported in the May 2009 edition of the International Journal of Clinical Practice. According to the research team of the University of Ioannina in Greece, excessive consumption of colas tends cause hypokalaemia or dangerously low blood potassium levels.

According to Dr Moses Elisaf, the author of the research paper, this condition could be triggered either by the fructose and caffeine in colas, or both ingredients. The study suggests that caffeine was the main culprit, though fructose is also suspect due to its tendency to cause diarrhea.

Chronic cola drinkers who have the following conditions are especially vulnerable to a shift in the electrolyte imbalance that low potassium levels entail: cardiac ischaemia, heart failure and left ventricular hypertrophy.

I have elaborated on why caffeine is a neurotoxin later in this book (Chapter 12: Energize, Not Exercise). Here is more bad news. Chronic cola drinkers are also susceptible to caffeine intoxication, which is characterized by a state of nervousness, anxiety, restlessness, insomnia, tremors, rapid heartbeat or tachycardia, restlessness and pacing, and in rare cases, death.

Sugar & Genes: Scientists may have unraveled a wealth of detail about the human body when the results of the Human Genome Project were announced in 2003. But the double helix that encodes the species' genetic information is still far from being fully understood.

For instance, researchers with Australia's Baker IDI Heart and Diabetes Institute announced in January 2009 that when the body experiences a 'sugar hit', as it does every time you drink a can of cola or when you consume a processed meal, your genes remember the event for up to two weeks.

The researchers, whose results were published in the Journal of Experimental Medicine, explain that a sudden intake of refined sugar or HFCS alters the body's natural metabolic processes that tend to otherwise protect the body against diabetes and heart disease.

According to the study, these changes last long after the actual 'hit' takes place at the genetic level, and if unhealthy dietary patterns continue, they could permanently alter human DNA.

The study relates to what researchers in the field of epigenetics have suspected for a while - that our genes provide us with the basic template that makes us human. But genetic expression, or the way your genes express themselves, can be altered by factors in your environment such as diet, chronic stress, sleeping habits and even the way you think.

Sweet Tooth, Sweet Tongue? You've probably heard the cliché about having a sweet tooth. But researchers at Penn State College of Medicine are now suggesting that obese individuals, at least some obese individuals, may have a 'sweet tongue'.

The researchers, whose findings were published in the Journal of Neurophysiology in November 2008, studied taste sensitivity in lean and obese rats.

They did this by observing differences in processing taste in the Pontine Parabrachial Nucleus or the part of the brain that uses nerve cells to relay information from the surface of the tongue to the brain.

They found that rats who were obese displayed varying sensitivity levels to varying concentrations of sucrose. When they were fed low to moderate levels of sucrose, the nerves (taste buds) on their tongues displayed only half the sensitivity to the sugar than lean rats. But when fed higher concentrations of sucrose, their tongues were more sensitive to the sugar than the lean rats were.

The researchers concluded that the obese rats, when fed low to medium concentrations of sucrose craved it because the 'sweet signal' from their tongues was too weak for their brains to perceive it. As a result, the brain and therefore the rat needed to consume more sucrose before the brain could decide that the body had had enough.

What does this mean for human beings? Most processed foods, which contain HFCS and refined sugar, are not terribly sweet, to the taste buds, at least. Like the rats, could the tongues of obese individuals, too, be less sensitive to sucrose, pushing them to eat more of these foods before the brain finally gets the message?

This hypothesis relates to another issue with obesity. Dopamine levels are usually lower than normal in obese individuals. Dopamine is the neurotransmitter that activates the reward or 'pleasure' centre of the brain.

When dopamine levels are low, overweight individuals tend to eat more foods that they enjoy (read processed and sweet foods and sugary drinks) to feel 'fully satisfied'.

This contributes to chronic consumption of foods and beverages that promote obesity, and further relates to issues such as insulin and leptin resistance.

Does this mean that obese individuals have fewer taste buds or defective taste buds? Some researchers have found that leptin, the hormone produced by the body's fat cells and controls the satiety response, binds to taste receptors on the tongue.

A large percentage of overweight individuals are also leptin resistant, which means that the brain's satiety signals are malfunctioning and the brain is unable to turn off your appetite when your blood glucose levels rise.

Hence, the decreased sensitivity to sugar and processed foods may not be a deficiency in taste per se but the result of leptin resistance.

Food Labels: Sweet Confusion

Just when the sugar lobby had thought they had finally won their legendary battle with the corn lobby in 2008, the latter used the good offices of the FDA to extract sweet revenge. But since when has the FDA been an impartial referee in the battle for supremacy on food labels - or for the American palate and wallet?

Manufacturers of processed foods, the sugar lobby and the corn lobby have collectively conned the American public into quite literally buying a pack of lies for several decades.

One of the major prizes in the struggle for space on food labels is cornering the word 'natural'. Given the growing awareness among the American public about the damaging effects of processed foods, food manufacturers have been trying to 'return to nature' and turn 'all-natural', on food labels, at least.

With organic, natural foods growing in popularity, both the sugar and corn lobbies have been claiming that refined sugar and HFCS are 'natural sweeteners'.

Manufacturers of refined sugar have been claiming for a while now that the ingredient is 'made from natural ingredients'. Read carefully, and you will notice that this statement is both true and false.

Refined sugar, stripped of 90 percent of cane and beet and every trace of vitamins and minerals, is indeed made from natural ingredients - cane or beet. But with smart advertising, the sugar lobby has managed to convince us that 'refined' sugar *is* natural.

Miffed with all the attention sugar has been getting over the years, the Corn Refiners Association, launched a multi-million dollar advertising campaign in 2008 to whitewash the image of its much-maligned high-fructose corn syrup and its causal link to obesity.

With the tagline 'And Now A Little Food for Thought', the association spent $20 to $30 million on the campaign, including full-page advertisements in more than a dozen major newspapers, claiming that HFCS "is no worse for you than sugar".

This, despite the fact that corn growers receive around $40 billion in federal subsidies so that corn syrup remains the preferred sweetener over cane sugar.

But, it seems, the sugar lobby was able to successfully strike back, with some of the biggest food manufacturers replacing HFCS with old-fashioned sugar in their products and using this as a selling point.

For instance, ConAgra now uses only sugar or honey in its Healthy Choice All Natural frozen entrées, and Kraft Foods has removed HFCS from its salad dressings. Pizza Hut and Pepsi too have removed HFCS from some of their products and replaced it with sugar.

This coincides with two major advertising campaigns, one in 2003 and the other in 2007, launched by the Sugar Association, to promote sugar, you guessed it, as a 'natural' ingredient.

The campaigns, supported by more than a dozen sugar companies, were called 'Sugar, Sweet by Nature', which attempted to point out that sugar is found in fruits and vegetables and is hence natural.

The first campaign was launched in 2003, after three decades during which HFCS had been steadily replacing sugar in the American diet. Consumption of the two sweeteners finally drew even in 2003 (according to the US Department of Agriculture), sparking yet another round of rivalry.

So what constitutes 'natural', according to the FDA? According to the agency, "a 'natural' product is one that has not had any artificial or synthetic substances added to the product that would not normally be expected to be in the food -including artificial flavors or color additives, regardless of source."

In other words, the FDA does not restrict the use of the term 'natural' except on products that contain added color, synthetic substances and flavors *(as per Title 21 of the Code of Federal Regulations, Section 101.22)*

There are several problems with the two above-mentioned paragraphs, the main issue simply being how vague they are. After all, though there is nothing natural about refined sugar and HFCS, they are neither food coloring agents nor flavoring agents.

Yet, in April 2008, the FDA made a surprising comment, stating that HFCS is not 'natural'. The agency had received two petitions - one from the Sugar Association and the other from the bakery firm Sara Lee - but had replied to neither.

Then, in response to a petition from a nutrition website, Geraldine June, Supervisor of the Product Evaluation and Labeling team at the FDA's Office of Nutrition, Labeling and

Dietary Supplements, said: *"We would object to the use of the term 'natural' on a product containing HFCS because it is produced using synthetic fixing agents. The use of synthetic fixing agents in the enzyme preparation, which is then used to produce HFCS, would not be consistent with our (...) policy regarding the use of the term 'natural'."*

Just when the Sugar Association was celebrating, the FDA did an inexplicable flip-flop just three months later. This was after the rival Corn Refiners Association demanded that the FDA further clarify its stand. The agency cleverly issued a statement.

Backtracking on the statement she had made three months earlier, Geraldine June said that when HFCS is made using the process presented by Archer Daniels Midland Company, the sweetener can be considered 'natural'.

This process sees the enzymes to make HFCS being fixed to a column by the use of a synthetic fixing agent called glutaraldehyde. However, this agent does not come into contact with the high dextrose equivalent corn starch hydrolysate and so it is not *"considered to be included or added to the HFCS,"* June 'clarified'.

She added: *"However, we would object to the use of the term 'natural' on a product containing HFCS that has a synthetic substance such as a synthetic fixing agent included in or added to it."*

Cornering the market share for a 'natural' sweetener is a billion-dollar dog-fight and both sugar millers and corn growers have very deep pockets. The question therefore is: Does the FDA, tasked with protecting the American consumer from dangerous ingredients included by food manufacturers, have the moral right to deliberately confuse the population?

Chapter 8: Righting a Wrong

The Cholesterol Myth

How the pharmaceutical industry loves disease! Better still, it is especially gleeful about creating myths, carefully crafted ones, many of which have become the touchstones of modern medicine.

This is why most of us have come to fear the 'C' word - 'cholesterol'. We are told that cholesterol is bad for health and leads to obesity and various types of cardiovascular disease including cardiac arrest and stroke.

Next we are told that there are two types of cholesterol - 'good' cholesterol and 'bad' cholesterol. Then we are told that high cholesterol levels are the primary cause of heart disease.

And finally, the clincher. Modern medicine says that if your cholesterol levels are elevated, certain drugs will effectively lower these levels and thus greatly reduce your risk of heart disease.

Now what if I told you that much of this is actually not true? What if I said refined sugar, not cholesterol, was one of the main culprits of vascular and coronary disease?

But let us start at the very beginning. Let us start by breaking the association between cholesterol and heart disease, and explore the myths that have made cholesterol the 'bad guy' in obesity and coronary disease.

What Is Cholesterol? Cholesterol is a waxy, fatty substance that arises from two sources: the food you eat and your liver. Foods such as animal proteins, poultry and dairy products are good sources of cholesterol. The other source is the liver, which both manufacturers cholesterol when the body needs it and regulates the amount of cholesterol in your bloodstream.

Good Guy, Bad Guy: We have been told time and again that there are mainly two types of cholesterol - 'good' cholesterol and 'bad' cholesterol. This is untrue for two very good reasons. What we refer to as 'good' and 'bad' cholesterol are actually High-Density Lipoprotein (HDL) and Low-Density Lipoprotein (LDL).

HDL and LDL are *not* cholesterol. They are protein molecules that bind with cholesterol and transport it from the liver via the bloodstream to the trillions of cells in the human body. Cholesterol needs this transport system because it is fatty and does not mix well with water-based blood.

LDL is much-maligned because modern medicine has made us believe that it sticks to the walls of the arteries and causes plaque to accumulate. On the other hand, we have been told that HDL is 'good' because it has the ability to dislodge the LDL from the arteries and transport it back to the liver, where it is recycled.

The fact is that neither LDL nor HDL is good or bad. Cholesterol is a basic component of the body's cell membranes or cell walls. It is needed to build and repair the membranes, and keep them permeable and fluid. It is also important for the production and synthesis of bile acids, steroid hormones, and several fat-soluble vitamins. Cholesterol is the 'good guy', not the 'bad'.

Insulin and Leptin: Insulin and leptin are two hormones produced by two very different organs of the body - the pancreas and adipose tissue, respectively. While insulin controls blood sugar levels, leptin helps regulate appetite by triggering the satiety response when your body has eaten sufficient food.

Individuals who are overweight or obese and those who are diabetic are often insulin and leptin resistant. This triggers a self-perpetuating and self-defeating loop that results in more weight gain and exacerbates obesity.

How are these hormones linked to cardiovascular disease? Studies have demonstrated that insulin and leptin resistance results in the formation of a large number of 'small dense' LDL particles. These microscopic LDL particles squeeze between the cells inside the lining of the arteries, or the 'gap junction' of the endothelium.

Once lodged here, these particles tend to oxidize and turn rancid. This causes the insides of the arterial walls to get inflamed and accumulate scars or plaque.

That is why it is important for all types of cholesterol to keep circulating in the blood, allowing the liver to regulate their levels. (Remember, if you eat a balanced diet and exercise regularly, your body will self-regulate)

It is therefore not the cholesterol itself that places you at cardiovascular risk. It is a defect in insulin and leptin signaling, which causes the cholesterol to oxidize and the liver, which manufactures the cholesterol, to malfunction.

Lowering your cholesterol levels will therefore do little to improve your health. Alternatively, identifying and addressing the underlying cause of inflammation will restore you to good health.

Lowering your cholesterol levels is meaningless for another reason. LDL particles come in many sizes, and large LDL particles do not cause problems. It is the small, dense LDL particles that can potentially cause inflammation.

So there you have it - 'good' LDL and 'bad' LDL, not 'good' cholesterol and 'bad' cholesterol!

Also, studies have shown that HDL particles too are rather differentiated, with some being better than others. That is why knowing your total cholesterol level, or even LDL and HDL levels, does not tell you anything at all!

Insulin and leptin have been more obviously linked to obesity and diabetes. Now it is clear that they also play a pivotal role in atherosclerosis and heart disease.

Inflammation & Heart Disease: Even though there are numerous causes of cardiovascular disease, the pharma industry and most doctors ignore them while choosing to point an accusing finger at cholesterol.

The fact is that if you are overweight or obese, chances are that the levels of various bio-chemicals, hormones and neurotransmitters in your body are also far from normal. This, by default, includes cholesterol, ingested as it is by a majority of individuals in the form of animal products, poultry and dairy products.

One reason could be fatty liver disease, a condition many obese individuals are afflicted with. (See Chapter 4: The Big Three). A fatty liver cannot adequately regulate cholesterol levels; neither can it perform the 500-odd functions it is tasked with.

So apart from assessing your cholesterol levels, have you ever tried to find out whether there is something else in your diet or lifestyle that is setting you up for a heart attack, a stroke or atherosclerosis? Have you ever wondered whether you are a victim of chronic inflammation which could be causing your arteries and heart to malfunction?

What Is Inflammation? Tissues get inflamed when they are damaged. Inflammation is a healing process whereby certain chemicals are released at the site of damage to repair the injured tissue. One of these chemicals is prostaglandins which promote inflammation, pain and fever and help the platelets in the blood to form a clot at the damaged site. Prostaglandins perform an important function unless the process that triggers their release is defective.

When tissue is damaged, the immune system also rushes white blood cells to the site to prevent harmful viruses and bacteria from invading it, and to consume and clean up the damaged debris.

Neighboring cells are also directed to multiply to repair the damage so that the tissue can heal. Not least of all, cholesterol is transported to the site of injury so that cells can repair themselves and rejuvenate.

Similar events take place within the lining of our arteries over a period of time, which leads to chronic, low-grade inflammation. When this happens, scars form in the lining of the arteries. This is called plaque. The result is constriction of the arteries, which sets the stage of high blood pressure and a heart attack. When this happens in the arteries supplying blood to the brain, it could lead to a stroke.

What causes our tissues to get chronically inflamed? Nature intended inflammation to be a temporary process, lasting only till the damaged tissues are repaired. Chronic inflammation is therefore not normal and may be caused by several factors.

Some of these are:
- Cigarette smoking
- Hypertension
- Lipoproteins
- Hyperglycemia

All these factors are believed to release chemicals that activate the cells involved in the inflammatory process.

Not only do they contribute to the formation of plaque in the arteries, they sometimes lead to the formation of blood clots in the arteries. These clots form when the inner linings of the arteries are damaged and bleed.

Chronic, low-grade infection may also lead to atherosclerosis. In fact, studies have found that the chlamydia pneumoniae bacterium and the herpes simplex virus are closely linked to the formation of atherosclerotic plaque.

Sugar, Not Cholesterol: It is no secret that refined sugar is a leading cause of obesity. An increasing body of research is now unraveling its role in inflammation and heart disease in ways you never suspected.

Apart from a host of other ill-effects, sugar - glucose and especially fructose - causes chronic damage to the body's cells through a process called glycation.

This is a biochemical process whereby either glucose or fructose molecules attach themselves to protein or fat. The byproducts of this process are called Advanced Glycation End Products or AGEs, which cause damage within the body's cells, and consequently, tissue inflammation.

Glycation can take place outside the body, for instance, by adding sugar to hot French fries or baked goods to enhance browning. The food processing industry has been using AGEs as flavor enhancers and coloring agents for 50 years to brown or caramelize products such as donuts, barbecued meats, cake and dark soda pop.

Glycation takes place inside the body as well, when you consume too much fructose and glucose. It disrupts molecular and cellular functioning across the body and releases highly-oxidizing AGEs such as hydrogen peroxide.

Some AGEs are benign but many damage endothelial tissue, fibrinogen and collagen in the cells across the body and give rise to diseases such as Alzheimer's, cancer, peripheral neuropathy, deafness, and blindness due to microvascular damage in the retina.

They have been causally linked to age-related chronic diseases such as type 1 and type 2 diabetes, cardiovascular disease and atherosclerosis.

Glycation and the formation of AGEs have been consistently found in individuals suffering from diabetes. Many diabetic patients, who are by definition insulin-resistant, suffer from hyperglycemia.

Unless introduced through diet, AGEs accumulate in the body when the body is unable to regulate its blood sugar levels. This is usually the case with obese individuals, who are often insulin and leptin resistant.

When blood sugar levels are abnormally elevated - because insulin is no longer doing its job - glucose levels could rise within the cells. This causes havoc, including the formation of AGEs inside the cells. What you are left with is massive cell and tissue damage across the body, including the insides of your arteries.

As explained above, when AGEs affect the interior of the arterial walls, it causes plaque to form. This tends to occur in areas of high blood flow such as the entrance to the coronary arteries.

Glycation has also been observed to stiffen collagen in the arteries, leading to high blood pressure. It could also lead to micro- or macro-aneurisms and strokes when this occurs in the brain.

What Are Statins? If your cholesterol level is higher than it should be, you should avoid taking statins.

Drugs containing statins, widely prescribed to lower cholesterol, accounted for $14.5 billion in sales in 2008 alone. They inhibit an enzyme that manufactures cholesterol in the liver. But they do much more than that.

There is an overwhelming body of evidence which shows that drugs that contain statins:

- Cause muscle pain and weakness due to the activation of atrogin-1, a gene which plays a role in muscle atrophy
- Precipitate a life-threatening condition called rhabdomyolysis, which causes your muscle cells to break down (In 2001, cerivastatin (Baycol) was withdrawn from the market after it was linked to rhabdomyolysis in patients)
- Inhibit a vital enzyme that manufactures cholesterol in the liver. It also inhibits another enzyme called 'Coenzyme Q10' whose depletion leads to muscle fatigue and weakness, soreness, and the breakdown of skeletal muscle tissue. In some cases, this could lead to congestive heart failure. Coenzyme Q10 is

especially vital to heart health as it supplies cellular energy to the organ.

Isn't it ironic that a drug that apparently protects you from cholesterol-induced heart disease can potentially - and fatally - damage your heart muscle?

How Low Is Too Low? Let me tell you the real truth about statins. But first, the facts. Till 2004, the acceptable level of cholesterol was pegged at 130 milligrams of LDL cholesterol. In that year, suddenly and inexplicably, the US Government's National Cholesterol Education Program advised patients at risk of heart disease to reduce their cholesterol levels to as little as 100 or even 70.

Clearly, it is impossible to achieve this ridiculous target without taking drugs (read statins). In one clever stroke, the revised guidelines therefore further opened up the market for this class of drugs, whose popularity was already on the rise.

The US Government couldn't have timed its advice any better. According to data released by another arm of the US Government - the US Agency for Healthcare Research and Quality - the use of statins rose by 156 percent between 2000 and 2005, while spending catapulted from $7.7 billion to $19.7 billion during this period.

As for the number of Americans using statins, the figure rose from 15.8 million to 29.7 million between 2000 and 2005.

Now here is the bitter truth about the revised guidelines released by the National Cholesterol Education Program.

Eight of the nine doctors on the panel were financially linked to companies manufacturing those cholesterol-lowering drugs. Two of them owned stock in these companies, two others were appointed to drug companies after working on these guidelines, and one doctor was a senior government scientist who was associated with ten drug companies.

Here is another bitter pill. Research studies that promote a specific drug or class of drugs, including statins, are almost always funded by a pharmaceutical company with vested interests in the results (as the notorious JUPITER trials showed). That should tell you to enough to be wary of what you read and what the media publishes.

If the drug companies, the doctors on their payrolls and the media could have their way, they would have your cholesterol levels see-sawing, depending on the advice they dole out from time to time.

What they won't tell you is that low cholesterol levels raise your risk of:

- nerve damage
- memory loss
- cancer
- Parkinson's disease
- depression
- aggression and violent behavior
- suicide

If the level of cholesterol in your bloodstream is indeed consistently elevated, you might want to consider the fact that chronic inflammation might be causing it. They may be high because when your cells get damaged, cholesterol is being transported to these sites to repair the damage. So it is not your cholesterol level you need to address but the reasons why there is so much of it in circulation.

Here are some common culprits of chronic inflammation:

- A diet high in refined sugar and grains
- Too many processed foods
- Animal proteins (See 'The Secret Cause Of Heart Disease - And Why It's So Easily Reversed' in *Timeless Secrets of Health and Rejuvenation*)
- Inactivity and lack of exercise
- Chronic emotional stress
- Smoking

It might take a while but simple lifestyle and dietary changes will help bring your insulin and leptin levels, among other biochemical processes, under control. These are triggers for inflammation and correcting the imbalance will restore your body to health.

Before I conclude, I would like to briefly recap the myths - and the reality - surrounding cholesterol.

Myth No 1: "Cholesterol is bad." Cholesterol is critical for the nervous system. It is essential for the growth and regeneration of the myelin sheath, or the sheath that covers the nerves and facilitates the conduction of electrical impulses. Cholesterol is also essential for the synthesis of bile, steroid hormones and fat-soluble vitamins

Myth No 2: "Cholesterol causes cardiovascular disease." It doesn't. Inflammation does

Myth No 3: "There's 'good' and 'bad' cholesterol." Cholesterol is the 'good guy'. As long as it keeps circulating, it does not cause damage. Inflammation is the 'bad guy'.

Myth No 4: "It is important to lower cholesterol levels." Cholesterol 'level' is meaningless. What matters is the type and number of cholesterol particles in the blood.

Chapter 9: Master Fixers

Enzymes: Nature's Catalysts

Digestion is one of the master keys to good health. And making digestion possible is a host of enzymes, most of them made and secreted by the liver, pancreas and small intestine.

These organs, along with the stomach, form the bulk of the digestive tract, which is where toxicity crises originate. That is why the key to good health is not only eating right but also creating the conditions for proper digestion. This makes sure that the food you eat actually nourishes your body.

At the centre of your digestive processes are different types of enzymes, which break down the main food groups - carbohydrates, proteins, fats and fiber - into smaller, digestible components. Enzymes further help the blood, organs, tissues and cells to absorb these nutrients and use them to burn fuel to stay alive, repair themselves, reproduce, and fight off pathogens.

But enzymes - many of them are not directly concerned with digestion - do a lot more. They help the body to use the vitamins and minerals you ingest, they synthesize and regulate hormones, they are vital to the health of your immune system, and they assist in detoxification processes. Each of these systems and processes is either directly or indirectly connected to weight loss.

The tricky part is making sure your digestive processes are always fine-tuned. It is therefore vital that your liver functions at optimal capacity because the liver produces bile, perhaps the most important natural facilitator for metabolism.

Though bile is manufactured in the liver, it is stored in the gall blabber, from where it is released into the small intestine as and when required. It not only metabolizes food but also works in tandem with each of the other digestive organs. It triggers the release of acids and enzymes from them, synthesizes enzymes with the help of the chemicals they release, and combines with their enzymes in perfect synchronization.

For instance, when you put a morsel of food in your mouth, the liver instantly prepares the way for digestion. Bile flows out of the gall bladder and pours into the common bile duct. This activates pancreatic enzymes, which are essential for the proper digestion of food. The bile then combines with these enzymes in the small intestine to metabolize food.

Bile and the digestive enzymes also work closely with stomach acid to provide the best possible basis for effective digestion of food. When one of these is under- or over-produced, the body automatically adjusts the production of the others to avoid further complications.

For example, if bile secretion is inadequate and, therefore, fewer pancreatic enzymes are activated, the stomach will reduce the secretion of hydrochloric acid (HCl) as well.

Otherwise, the alkaline bile and pancreatic juices will not be able to neutralize all the HCl as it enters the duodenum along with the food. This could cause ulcers in the duodenum and inflammation throughout the gastrointestinal tract.

There is basically no shortcut to achieving good digestive functions without sufficient and balanced bile secretions. Therefore, instead of supplementing with enzymes or HCl, it is best to clean out the liver and gall bladder.

In addition, you should take care that the other factors that control good digestion are also present. These would include masticating food thoroughly which stimulates the production of digestive enzymes both in the mouth and in the pancreas, eating the main meal of the day when secretion of digestive juices peaks around noon, avoiding eating food after 7 pm when digestive secretions drop dramatically, sleeping before 10 pm to provide the liver with enough energy and blood to produce enough bile to last for the following day, and of course eating a diet that is balanced and contains foods that are natural and do not require too much effort to digest them.

Some foods are naturally rich in enzymes and there is a sufficient variety. These include pineapple, avocado, grapes, papaya, and soaked or sprouted nuts and seeds. After you begin to incorporate enzyme-rich foods into your diet, your appetite and energy levels may take a couple of weeks to adjust. After that, you will experience a perceptible change in your health.

Think of it this way. One of the liver's most important functions is to break down toxins and prepare them for elimination. When disease sets in, the liver's capacity to detoxify the body is compromised, and a body that has been consistently undernourished is now being cleansed and re-adjusted.

The greater the toxic build-up and the longer you have been feeding your body processed foods and creating an unhealthy internal environment, the greater the adjustment it has to make. Healing takes a while but it is a lasting route to natural weight loss.

Let us examine the role of bile and three natural enzymes, all of them produced by the body and at the centre of the digestive process. This will give you an idea of just how complex the roles of bile and the main digestive enzymes - protease, amylase and lipase - are.

Bile: Bile is composed of bile acids, bile salts, cholesterol, water and bile pigments. Considering its multiple functions and how central the liver is to your overall health, I cannot stress how important it is for bile secretions to be normal.

Let me outline the main functions of this natural facilitator.

- Bile stimulates the production of pancreatic enzymes.
- Bile acids are critical for the digestion, transport and absorption of fat-soluble vitamins. Along with lipase from the pancreas, they assist in the digestion, transport and absorption of fat-soluble nutrients released from triglycerides ingested in your diet.
- Bile metabolizes toxins, including the metabolites released by the action of pharmaceutical drugs in the

body. It then prepares these toxic metabolites for elimination in the feces.

- Bile is an alkaline solution and keeps the internal environment of the small intestine alkaline to neutralize the vast quantities of HCL secreted by the stomach into the duodenum.
- Bile enjoys a reciprocal relationship with cholesterol, which it both digests for absorption by the bloodstream as well as requires for the manufacture of bile acids by the liver.
- For cholesterol to be digested, it must first be emulsified. In an action similar to detergents, bile acids break down fat globules into tiny droplets. This increases the surface area of fat, making it possible for lipase secreted by the pancreas to further metabolize it.
- Bile is also a lipid carrier, without which metabolized fatty acids, cholesterol and triglycerides cannot be transported in the bloodstream.

Protease: Protease is actually a group of enzymes that break down or hydrolyze proteins in the food you eat. Proteins are broken down into chains of molecules called amino acids, which are the fundamental building blocks of every cell in your body.

In the digestive tract, protease enzymes break the peptide bonds in protein foods to free the amino acids.

These enzymes also play an important role in the immune system. The digestive tract is often clogged with masses of undigested proteins. This is especially true if you eat a lot of animal protein or red meats, a dietary choice of many overweight individuals.

Protease enzymes also break down undigested protein, cellular debris, and toxins in the blood, which leaves the immune system free to perform its basic function of protecting your body against pathogens such as bacteria, viruses and other parasites.

When your pancreas cannot manufacture sufficient protease enzymes, it leads to an imbalance in the delicate acid-alkaline ratio in the small intestine since foods rich in proteins, especially animal proteins, lead to acidity, insomnia and anxiety.

Our bodies also need protein to transport protein-bound calcium in the blood. A protease deficiency could mean arthritis, osteoporosis and other diseases arising out of calcium deficiency.

Amylase: Amylase is another natural enzyme made by the pancreas. It is also secreted by the salivary glands in the mouth. If your body couldn't produce amylase, you would not be able to digest carbohydrates. Amylase breaks down the starch and sugar in carbohydrates into glucose, the fuel that powers every cell in your body.

Amylase also digests dead white blood cells. A lymphatic system deficient in amylase cannot effectively get rid of this debris, making you susceptible to pus formation.

Individuals who are deficient in amylase are prone to abscesses, which are inflamed pockets of tissue filled with pus. This invites bacteria and other parasites to these sites. This causes infection and further inflammation and the release of histamines.

The inflammatory response usually occurs in organs such as the lungs and skin, which are in contact with the outside environment. That is why some lung problems including asthma and emphysema may require amylase plus other enzymes to help them subside.

Lipase: Lipase is the third natural enzyme that is critical to digestion. It breaks down lipids or fats, cholesterol and triglycerides.

The key to fat digestion is a process called emulsification. Since fats are not water soluble, they cannot be transported through our watery blood and need to be made water-soluble first. This process of emulsification, or breaking down of large fat molecules into smaller, water-soluble globules, takes place mainly in the small intestine.

Triglycerides are emulsified by both bile and lipase, which work together in perfect synchronization in the lumen of the small intestine. After triglycerides are broken down or hydrolyzed into monoglycerides and fatty acids, the fat-soluble nutrients from the fats are absorbed into the bloodstream with the help of lipase and bile salts.

Lipase deficiency naturally leads to weight gain. The undigested fats are then stored in your adipose tissue in various sites across your body. It also leads to an increase in cholesterol and triglyceride levels.

Lipase is also required for the digestion of fat-soluble vitamins. Since it binds with the coenzyme chloride, lipase-deficient individuals tend to also have low chlorides in their electrolyte balance which is critical to the electrical activity in your nervous system.

Fats are also central to the health of every single one of your body's cells. If you are lipase-deficient, chances are your cell membranes are not as permeable as they should be. This means your cells are unable to absorb the nutrients they require and cannot excrete the waste material produced in them.

Is Raw More Healthy?

If processed foods are so damaging to our bodies, are uncooked or unprocessed foods the answer? Before I answer that question, here is something to think about. Did you know that when you heat food that is heated above 188 degrees Fahrenheit, the enzymes in it break down and are rendered useless?

In fact, the structure of the molecules changes completely, rendering the food inert and devoid of its life force. In other words, when you overcook food, you are actually killing its life force or Prana.

Processed foods are no different. They too are devoid of their life force and are nutritionally empty. That's why refined carbohydrates - such as refined flour, wheat and pasta, to name a few - are nutritionally deficient even though they add calories to your body. These are therefore called 'empty calories'.

Processed foods and overheated foods, when ingested, are interpreted by the body as pathogens or invaders as they are alien to its biochemistry. They instantly trigger the stress response and the immune system immediately releases white cells to 'fight the invader'.

Scientists who discovered this phenomenon back in the 1930s called this 'digestive leukocytosis' or a response of the leukocytes to a digestive process.

The logical conclusion is that eating foods in their raw and natural form is the healthiest way to eat. Or is it?

Many people who start on a raw, whole-food diet have already suffered from health problems and have weak Agni or digestive fire. Unable to break down the high food fiber, the intestinal bacteria start taking over that job. This results in fermentation and putrefaction of the food.

The poison, which the bacteria produce during the fermenting process, greatly stimulates the immune system and helps the body to dispose of it. This strong cleansing reaction initially helps clear the intestines of impacted fecal matter, stops constipation, and through the intense immune activity releases plenty of energy.

The relief from congestion and constipation and the increased energy and vitality are perceptible and strikes one as very a 'positive sign'. This response can even lead to a spontaneous remission of cancer or the relief of arthritic pains. But eventually, the intestines may begin to bloat like a balloon, unable to deal with the toxic gases and poisonous compounds.

Young Pitta types with a strong Agni and plenty of exercise can cope with a diet of raw foods for many years without harmful side-effects. But eventually, even their digestive system may become exhausted because of trying to break down these vegetables and grains.

Alternatively, Vata types and Kapha types may suffer ill-effects within days or weeks. These two types benefit more from eating mostly warm and cooked foods, as their bodies tend to be cool by nature.

A Kapha's Agni may easily get subdued by a lot of raw food, and a Vata, whose Agni is changeable, could become constipated, nervous, and depressed if he or she eats too much of it.

Here is why eating raw foods consistently weakens your digestive system and eventually leads to fatigue. It is not always easy to use the enzymes inside the cells of plant foods. The harder vegetables contain indigestible fiber consisting of cellulose which is the cell membrane. Softer vegetables like lettuce, avocado, tomatoes, basal, cilantro, cucumber, etc have very thin cell membranes which break down during the mastication process.

The tough cell membranes of harder vegetables remain intact if eaten raw (think of chewing on a carrot), making it relatively difficult for the body to digest and assimilate the nutrients.

If eaten in large amounts, they produce gas, the result of destructive fermentation. If cooked, the cell membranes break down and the nutrients can be digested and absorbed.

Contrast this with the cow, which has three stomachs that serve as cooking devices which, with the help of heat, bacteria and moisture, soften up and break down the cell membranes in plant foods.

Since humans do not have this ability, we may need to use heat and other food preparation methods such as fermenting foods (cultured foods), even if it destroys some of the enzymes and vitamins in the process.

Cooking harder plants foods also helps to eliminate natural antibodies which otherwise may cause irritation in the gut. For these reasons, food preparation has been an essential part of every ancient civilization, such as the Vedic, Mayan, Greek and Egyptian civilizations.

That does not mean you must altogether eliminate raw food from your diet. Eating salads, for instance, is a very healthy practice. Make it part of your afternoon meal and include raw vegetables as they contain healthy amounts of minerals and vitamins, proteins and fiber - all in their natural form. (Organic vegetables are recommended because commercially grown vegetables are treated with insecticides and other chemicals)

As mentioned earlier, your body type plays an important part in determining whether and how much raw salad you can tolerate. Whatever body type you are, also start trusting your intuition and listening to the signals your body sends out.

If you ate a salad or fruit for supper, you may feel sluggish and irritable the next morning because it has fermented in your intestines during the night. Nobody knows your body better than you do.

Also, if you feel inclined to only eating raw, unprepared foods, it means your body may require cleansing. Still, keep listening to your body's signals of comfort and discomfort. If one day you get an aversion to these foods, return to a mixed diet immediately because your body is telling you that it has had enough and can no longer cope with so many toxic and irritating antigens.

A cleanse consisting of raw vegetables or their juices has saved many people's lives by triggering a strong immune response. This helped remove toxic waste that may have lingered in the intestinal tract for many years. The body usually sends a clear message of discomfort when the antibodies begin to damage the intestines, which means it is time to stop the cleansing.

Here is a tip when eating salad. Always eat it at the beginning of your meal, before eating any cooked food. Since raw foods require different digestive enzymes than those needed for digesting cooked foods, eating these food items one after the other makes it easier on the digestive system.

Also, always eat raw foods at the beginning of a meal, not once you have eaten cooked food. Eating raw food items after having eaten cooked foods will leave them mostly undigested and subject to fermentation. Avoid cooked foods items in your salad, especially protein foods.

Eating the Rainbow

If you are trying to lose weight, you have probably heard it again and again: "Try eating fruits and vegetables." Conventional wisdom is usually right. Fruits and vegetables help you lose weight for a variety of reasons. But let us examine the simplest, most logical reasons, the ones that usually elude most of us!

It is all packed into one simple phrase: 'energy density'. Energy density is the amount of energy or number of calories that are packed into a unit of food (or a given volume). Let us call that a 'serving' or 'portion'.

Meat is energy-dense because it packs a large number of calories into a small portion. Fatty foods are even more energy dense. The least energy-dense foods are fruits and vegetables.

That is because they have very high water content. They are also high in fiber - and neither water nor fiber contains calories. Fruits and vegetables are therefore 'high-volume foods'.

This means you need to eat a larger portion of fruit and vegetables than meat to consume the same number of calories.

When you compare one serving of vegetable to a serving of meat, you get significantly less calories in the serving of vegetables. Now you are probably thinking you need to eat more vegetables to get the same number of calories that your usually meaty meal gives you, right? Wrong.

Human beings usually tend to eat a consistent quantity of food. Hence, when you consider volume alone, you need to eat more meat (and consume more calories) to 'feel full' as you would eat vegetables.

Let me put it another way. When you eat vegetables, you 'feel full' faster and on fewer calories! Simple, isn't it?

There is another reason why fruits and vegetables help you lose weight. They turn off food cravings. Processed foods, especially those high in refined sugars and carbohydrates, make the body crave for more. However, fruits and vegetables short circuit the food-addiction cycle.

Fruits and vegetables are nutrition powerhouses as they contain all the vitamins, minerals, enzymes, fiber, antioxidants and protein that the body requires. Unlike processed foods, which trick the body into believing it is full even when it has not received the nutrients it requires, fruits and vegetables are 'honest foods' as they provide it with all that is healthy. But you do have to eat a variety of them.

Isn't it shocking that the average American eats a diet containing only 8 percent of fruits and vegetables? If the other 92 percent consists of nutritionally empty foods, is it any wonder that food cravings and weight gain are widespread among the population?

You can start to eat healthy gradually, slowly increasing the fruit and vegetable content of your diet. Start with salads and soup and increase the vegetarian component while reducing meats and processed foods.

It won't be long before you notice the difference in your energy levels and weight too!

Now who doesn't feel like a good old snack every now and then? If you are keen to lose weight and give up potato chips, turkey sandwiches and nachos, here are some suggestions for tasty and nutritious snacks that *won't* make you pile on the pounds.

Dried fruit are an amazing snack with superlative health benefits. They are sweet and nutrient-dense, denser than when the fruit is fresh. They reduce the risk of cancer, provide an energy boost, lower blood pressure, lower the risk of cardiovascular disease, keep cholesterol in check, prevent diabetes, and thanks to the antioxidants in them, they slow the aging process.

Among dried fruit, almonds are an especially healthy choice, for several reasons. Here are some of them. Thanks to the generous amount of Vitamin E (which has antioxidant properties) in them, almonds lower the risk of cardiac problems. They are high on monounsaturated fats and hence they also lower LDL cholesterol levels.

This nut also contains magnesium and potassium. Magnesium helps the blood vessels to relax, allowing normal blood flow. Potassium helps in nerve transmission and is important to heart health.

Almonds also have the ability to stabilize blood sugar levels and prevent insulin spikes, which lead to food cravings and weight gain.

One study, published in the *International Journal of Obesity and Related Metabolic Disorders,* found that adding almonds to a low-calorie diet helps overweight individuals lose weight more effectively than a low-calorie diet high in complex carbohydrates.

The *Institute of Food Research* has published studies which found that almonds have prebiotic properties. These nuts provide nutrition for gut bacteria or 'friendly bacteria' so that they can flourish inside the intestines, thereby improving digestion and the immune system.

Another study, whose results were published in the *European Journal of Clinical Nutrition*, found that a diet that includes almonds lowers not only LDL cholesterol but also C-reactive protein levels. C-reactive protein is a key marker for inflammation, which leads to clogged arteries or atherosclerosis and heart disease.

Chapter 10: Coming Clean

Disease: The Ultimate Adjustment

The human body has an amazing capacity to adjust and absorb the abuse most of us subject it to. Such abuse consists of disastrous dietary habits (nutritional deficiencies, undernourishment, overeating and overdependence on processed foods), irregular eating habits, erratic sleep patterns (for party animals and frequent fliers, none at all!), too little activity or no exercise at all, and chronic stress, and all this takes a physical toll.

When we take our body for granted, its natural functions get distorted to accommodate our unmindful, even willful behavior. You would be more than a little surprised at the type and amount of debris you have accumulated inside your digestive and alimentary tracts.

What's more, most of us are not even aware of the undigested food, rotting meat, clogged metabolic poisons and calcified gallstones that are choking our internal organs and providing a fertile breeding ground for harmful bacteria.

Finally, when the body reaches its toxicity threshold, it enters a diseased state and signals that something is terribly wrong. While all diseases start with a toxicity crisis, the symptoms (what conventional medicine refers to as the disease) vary.

This is because different people have different physical vulnerabilities. That is why some individuals may develop an acute sensitivity to allergens or acne, others digestive disorders while still others may develop cancer.

The type of organ or system that gives in is usually the weakest and therefore the most vulnerable because it is least likely to fight back. The organ then begins to act as a defense system so that poisons are kept at bay and don't flood the bloodstream. If that were to happen, you would perish from toxic overload.

The course the disease takes will depend on which organ or system is affected but it all begins when the body is under toxic assault.

So just like diabetes, ulcers, vertigo, or asthma, obesity is also a toxicity crisis, where the body stores fat as a defense mechanism. As long as the reason exists, the body will *need* to put on weight. That is why dieting and exercising usually don't work.

It is an empirical fact that obese individuals have high levels of toxins stored in their fatty tissue. Adipose tissue has a relatively low level of metabolic activity, and storing poisons in the fatty deposits keeps them from entering the bloodstream and vital organs. The body is thus literally protecting itself from being poisoned.

Research has shown that when an individual's weight exceeds more than 20 pounds over their ideal body weight, adipose tissue begins to act like a separate endocrine organ. It begins to secrete hormones such as leptin and cortisol, which through complex biochemical processes encourage further fat storage.

Cortisol, apart from promoting insulin resistance, leads to the breakdown of proteins in muscles for conversion into glucose. Since many overweight individuals are insulin resistant, glucose, instead of being burned, is converted into fat.

So while your muscle mass decreases, body fat increases. This vicious cycle is very difficult to break and it's part of the reason why 'fat people seem to get fatter'.

Most toxins are physical by nature - processed foods, refined carbohydrates and sugars, chemical ingredients and preservatives in foods, high-fructose corn syrup, chemical pesticides and medical drugs. But toxins can also have an emotional origin.

Either due to temperament or traumatic events in one's past, an individual can become emotionally toxic. Old conflicts, traumas and toxic beliefs continue to rankle long after they have subsided from the conscious mind. These are stored as poisonous compounds in adipose or fatty tissue.

During the 37 years that I have practiced natural medicine, I have come across many jolly, happy-go-lucky obese men and women, none of whom had the slightest inkling that their bodies were a safe-house for old memories and traumas that they couldn't let go of.

Conventional medicine and weight-loss programs ignore anything they cannot see. So if you are overweight, it's got to be the unhealthy diet you are eating, or your sedentary lifestyle, or both.

While there is no denying that both these factors are crucial to any natural weight-loss plan, what I am trying to emphasize is that the conventional approach sidesteps the causes of disease while zeroing-in on symptoms.

Re-Balancing the Equation

Every cell in the body, and the body as a whole, is constantly striving to achieve a state of balance or equilibrium. An obese body is a body literally bending itself out of shape to defend itself from being poisoned. It is a body that is way out of sync with itself.

Everybody also has an optimal body weight, one where the individual is not warding off potential threats and poisons. Losing weight the natural way means reversing the processes that led to a state of toxicity. It also means simultaneously creating an environment that is conducive to vibrant health.

Re-balancing involves many things. It means the ability to let go of past traumas to improve blood and lymph circulation, raising immunity and restoring your internal organs to function as they were meant to.

It means healthy diet choices, getting sufficient sleep and at the right time, and detoxifying the body. During this purification process, the body is purged of toxins through a series of internal cleanses. It is therefore important to remember that losing weight is not a mechanical or mainly physical process.

Losing weight the natural way is a mental attitude that establishes an intimate connection between mind, body and spirit. This is the most effective and lasting way to regulate weight permanently.

Once you make that mental shift, just as your body once embraced a toxic state, it will now want to embrace good health and you will return to your natural weight. Once you go down this path, you will realize that there is no effort involved. It is a wanting that comes from within.

The best way to start re-balancing is to reverse the processes that led up to the toxic state. Obesity is a disease of stored body toxicity and before your body starts regulating itself, it needs to release the accumulated poisons.

This means detoxifying your body to cleanse yourself of the waste you have collected over the years. Weight regulation can start simultaneously, by re-balancing your lifestyle and beginning to incorporate healthy habits into your daily routine.

You may choose a pace that is comfortable for you, always keeping in mind that the more you are in tune with your body's innate wisdom and the closer you are to nature's rhythms (as close as modern urban life will allow), the sooner you will return to your optimal weight.

An effective natural way to cleanse and purify your body is to flush out poisons from your digestive tract and organs of elimination - the liver and gall bladder, small intestine, kidney, and colon or bowels.

Liver Flush: Flushing and cleansing these internal organs (Read more about this in my books *The Amazing Liver And Gallbladder Flush* and *Timeless Secrets of Health and Rejuvenation*) basically involves the use of natural substances such as apple juice, Epsom salts, olive oil and a little lemon juice.

What exactly do these ingredients do? Apple juice contains malic acid, which is a solvent and weakens the bonds between solid globules in the liver. Epsom salts or magnesium sulfate relaxes smooth muscle.

Hence, it both opens the bile ducts to facilitate the release of liquid bile for the flushing process and hardened stones from the gall bladder. Epsom salts also relaxes the bowel and facilitates bowel movement.

Unrefined olive oil makes the gall bladder and bile ducts contract and expel the gall stones.

If necessary, certain nutrients may be used to control and support the detoxification process. These supplements capture, isolate, and neutralize the toxins stubbornly stored in the body over the years and may include plant husk or fiber, especially fiber from fresh, raw fruits and vegetables.

Bentonite clay mixed with water may also be used as the molecules of the clay act as a natural sponge for the poisons flowing into the bloodstream. Another form of bentonite known as montmorillonite draws toxins out of the tissues.

The ingredients used vary depending on the therapist and individual's physiological needs and toxic state. But supervision is definitely advised. Some individuals have tried to cleanse their internal organs on advice from well-meaning friends and the Internet. Alas, many have suffered unnecessary complications.

Though the process itself is simple enough - a liver flush usually takes six days of preparation followed by 16 to 20 hours of actual cleansing - each individual may need the procedure to be customized according to their needs. This is best done under supervision.

There are also some precautions you need to take. Remember, flushing and cleansing the body releases poisons into the bloodstream. Just as these harmful chemical compounds would have destroyed your body if they were not stored, they could prove detrimental when released back into the bloodstream.

That is why when unsupervised, some individuals report experiencing symptoms such as fatigue, rashes, sinus congestion, fever, aches in the joints, flatulence and headaches. The more toxic the body, the greater the level of toxins released.

So how does internal cleansing assist in weight loss? In overweight individuals, the detoxification process releases fat stores. While excess fat is burned via metabolism, toxic material stored in the adipose tissue is transported to the liver. Here, it is broken down and prepared for excretion.

Also, enzyme and other pathways are cleared, allowing the internal organs to function as they were meant to. The immune system is also restored, and a re-balanced metabolism will ensure that the liver breaks down and neutralizes toxic chemicals in future. Of course, to keep your liver functioning normally, you will simultaneously need to eat healthy foods and possibly make some lifestyle changes.

Many overweight individuals also harbor a fatty liver. Once liver and gall bladder stones are flushed out, the liver can mobilize the glycogen or sugar that has remained stagnant inside it for years.

A reinvigorated liver will also be able to adequately process incoming fats while transporting excess lipids to the bowel for excretion. Also, since toxic stores of fat are being burned and the rest excreted, your metabolism will also be restored.

All this works in a loop and helps control blood sugar. This is because the body's hormonal balance is restored, and a body that is no longer overweight does not have to remain insulin resistant.

Although the liver flush on its own can produce truly amazing results, it should ideally be done after a kidney and colon cleanse. Cleansing the colon beforehand ensures that the expelled gallstones are easily removed from the large intestine

Cleansing the kidneys as well makes certain that toxins released by the liver during the liver flush do not overburden these vital organs of elimination. Also, make sure you cleanse your kidneys after every three liver flushes.

Hence, the most effective sequence is: kidneys cleanse - colon cleanse - liver flush - colon cleanse. It is important to repeat the liver flush at regular intervals until no more stones are being released. [For details on these cleanses, see *The Amazing Liver and Gallbladder Flush*]

Colonic Irrigation: Also called colon hydrotherapy or a colonic, colonic irrigation is perhaps one of the most effective colon cleansing therapies. Within a short period of time, a colonic can eliminate large amounts of trapped waste that may have taken many years to accumulate.

During a 40–50 minute session, two to six liters of distilled or purified water is used to gently flush the colon. Through a gentle abdominal massage, old deposits of mucoid fecal matter are loosened and subsequently flushed out by the water.

A colonic removes not only harmful, toxic waste, but it also tones, hydrates and rejuvenates the colon muscles. The repeated uptake and release of water improves the colon's peristaltic action and reduces the transit time of fecal matter.

In addition, colonic irrigation restores the colon's natural shape and stimulates the reflex points that connect the colon with other parts of the body. This form of colon cleansing can detach old crusted layers of waste from the walls of the large intestine, which permits better water absorption and hydration of the colon and the body as a whole.

However, it may take a minimum of two to three sessions to reap these benefits. After that, your bowel movements will be naturally restored in about two days.

If it takes longer, it indicates that the colon has accumulated unduly large amounts of waste over a period of time. To soften and flush it out may take a series of colonics and, of course, liver flushes, and a balanced diet and lifestyle.

Colonic irrigation can also help with emotional problems. It is no coincidence that the transverse colon passes right through the solar plexus, which is the body's emotional center. Most of our unresolved or 'undigested' emotional issues are stored in the solar plexus and result in tightening of the colon muscle. This may slow bowel movement and cause constipation.

Colonics can help clear the physical obstruction and release the tension that causes the emotional repression in the first place.

Kidney Cleanse: You may also need to cleanse the kidneys if the presence of gallstones in the liver, or other causes, have led to the development of stones in the kidneys or the urinary bladder.

The kidneys are very delicate, blood-filtering organs that are easily congested due to poor digestion, stress and an irregular lifestyle. The main causes of kidney congestion are stones. Most stones/crystals/sand, however, are too small to be recognized through modern diagnostic instruments such as X-rays.

Certain herbs, when taken daily for a period of 20–30 days, can help dissolve and eliminate all the various types of kidney stones, including uric acid stones, oxalic acid stones, phosphate stones and amino acid stones.

If you have a history of kidney stones and want to completely clean out these organs, you may want to repeat this cleanse several times, at intervals of six to eight weeks.

Ionized Water: Sipping hot ionized water has a profound effect on deep tissue-cleansing. It reduces overall toxicity, improves circulation and balances bile. When you boil water for 15 to 20 minutes, it becomes thinner (its molecule clusters are reduced from the usual 10,000 to one or two clusters), and it is charged and saturated with negative oxygen ions (hydroxide, OH^-).

When you take frequent sips of hot ionized water throughout the day, it begins to systematically cleanse the tissues of the body and help rid them of positively charged ions (those associated with harmful acids and toxins).

Most toxins and waste materials carry a positive charge and they naturally attach themselves to the body, which is overall negatively charged. As the negative oxygen ions enter the body with the ingested water, they are attracted to the positively charged toxic material. This neutralizes waste and toxins, turning them into fluid matter that the body can remove easily.

If you have excessive body weight, this cleansing method can help you shed many pounds of body waste in just weeks, without the side effects that normally accompany sudden weight loss.

Making ionized water is easy. All you have to do is boil water for 15 to 20 minutes and pour it into a thermos. The thermos keeps the water hot and ionized throughout the day. Take one or two sips every half hour all day long, and drink it as hot as you would sip tea.

Some individuals drink ionized water for a certain period of time, such as three to four weeks; others sip it every day.

This specially prepared water should not substitute for normal drinking water. It does not hydrate the cells like normal water does; the body uses it to only cleanse the tissues.

For weight loss to be permanent, cleansing and purifying the body needs to be accompanied by an attitudinal shift. The critical link here is the mind-body connection. Once this is established, you will naturally want to live healthy.

Losing weight will then be more than a healthy process you put your body through. Transcending cosmetic reasons, you will feel the need to rejuvenate and revitalize your energy and health.

Let me walk you through a ready reckoner of weight loss.

EATING

You have often heard the phrase "You are what you eat". And while that is true, it is only half the story. However, let us focus on dietary habits for the time being. What you eat, when you eat and how much you eat will determine the quality of nutrition your body gets.

Here are some quick pointers that will complement your overall weight-loss program.

Breakfast
Recommended

▶ Skipping breakfast is all right. Alternatively, eat a light breakfast, consisting of nutritious wholesome foods such as oatmeal (porridge) or any other hot cereal. A breakfast consisting of only fruit (other than citrus) is fine.

Avoid

▶ **Soy Milk**: Soy contains natural food toxins (enzyme inhibitors). It is also possibly genetically engineered and potentially affects hormonal balance.

▶ **Fruit With Cereals**: Avoid adding fruit to your cereals as this leads to fermentation and toxicity.

▶ **Animal Proteins**: Cheese, meat, ham or eggs as well as sour foods, including yogurt and citrus fruit quickly subdue Agni, or the digestive fire, which is naturally low in the morning.

Lunch
Recommended

▶ **When**: 12–12:30 pm (when the sun is in its highest position). Make lunch the main meal of the day.

Avoid

▶ **Beverages**: Liquids like alcohol and wine taken with meals dilute digestive juices and cause indigestion and weight gain.

Recommended

▶ **Water**: Sip a little hot water during your meal to increase your digestive power and maintain thinness of blood and normal secretions of bile. Also, drink a glass of water about 30 minutes before lunch and again two and a half hours after lunch.

▶ **Salads**: Raw and cooked foods require different digestive enzymes. Hence eat salad at the beginning of your meal. Eating raw foods after eating cooked foods will leave them undigested and subject to fermentation. As far as salad dressing goes, use a full-fat salad dressing, such as extra virgin olive oil and lemon juice. This helps digest raw salad.

Evening Meal

Recommended

▶ **When**: 6–7 pm (Agni is low at night. Eat an early dinner so that active digestion is completed before bedtime as the production of digestive enzymes stops at 8 pm)

▶ **Vegetables**: Eat freshly prepared vegetable soup, perhaps blended, served with whole wheat pita or spelt bread, whole wheat toast or rye crackers with unsalted butter, ghee or coconut oil.

Another option is cooked vegetables with rice or other light cooked grain foods. The soup/vegetables may be seasoned with spices and herbs, vegetable bouillon, unrefined sea salt, as well as butter, ghee or coconut oil added during or after cooking - about one teaspoon of butter, ghee or coconut oil per person (avoid other oils in the evening as they are more difficult to digest.

Avoid

▶ **Proteins**: Avoid meat, pork, poultry, fish, ham, eggs, nuts or any other concentrated form of protein because Agni is too low at this time to digest animal proteins.

▶ **Dairy Products**: Yoghurt, cheese, fruits and salads have naturally high bacteria content. They cause indigestion and fermentation at night.

▶ **Oily Foods**: Fried and deep-fried foods, as well as root vegetables such as potatoes (with the exception of cooked carrots, beets or white radishes), are also difficult to digest at night.

Remember, regularity is important: Regular meal times help the body know what and how much to expect. This avoids uncertainty, which the body interprets as a state of famine. This, in turn, prompts it to store glucose as fat and leads to weight gain.

Rules of Thumb

▶ Avoid **heavy foods**, oily and fried food, aged cheeses, yoghurt, onion and garlic.

▶ Include one or two pieces of **fresh fruit** per day in your diet. Drink only freshly prepared fruit juice (best diluted with water). Packaged juices are pasteurized and acid-forming. Many contain artificial sweeteners and should be avoided.

Fruit or fruit juices should always be taken on an empty stomach. The best times to eat fruit are mid-morning and mid-afternoon, or for breakfast with nothing else. Choose fruit that is in season and that which naturally grows in your environment.

▶ You may eat soaked **dry fruit**, eg, sultanas, figs, dates or prunes, either for breakfast (without other foods) or as a snack like other fruit. Soaking them makes them easily digestible.

▶ Eat 8–12 **almonds** (soaked and skinned) on a daily basis. They are good for the eyes and bones

▶ **Leftovers** are another no-no, with the exception of rice and beans. These may be refrigerated for a day or two.

▶ Another must-not-have is **frozen food**. It is devoid of the life force and thus has diminished nutrient-absorption.

▶ **Microwaves** used to cook food cause total disintegration of the food's molecular structure and destroy its life force. Microwave-cooked food is thus non-nutritious and thwarts digestion.

▶ **Ice-cold foods** or beverages 'extinguish' Agni for many hours. They may also numb and damage the nerve endings of the stomach, apart from making the stomach cells contract and preventing them from secreting the required amounts of digestive juices.

▶ Use **spices** appropriate for your body type generously. Spices not only enhance the flavor of food, but also contain vital nutrients and aromas that help with digestion and metabolism. Chili peppers or chili-containing spice mixes should be avoided, though, as they affect the chest and cause mucus irritation in the stomach and intestines.

▶ For one day per week or month, you may want to try taking only a **liquid diet** (soups, freshly made juices, water, herbal teas, ionized water, etc). Then gradually build up to a normal diet again. This relieves the strain on your digestive system and improves its ability to remove accumulated toxic waste.

At Mealtimes...

▶ Remain seated when you eat. The digestive system is better able to secrete balanced amounts of digestive juices when you are eating in the seated position.

▶ Eat in a peaceful environment without radio, television or reading. Any distraction from eating impairs the body's ability to supply the appropriate enzymes for digestion.

▶ Sit quietly for at least five minutes after the meal so that the food has a chance to settle in your stomach before you get up from the table. A short and leisurely walk after meals greatly aids digestion.

▶ Chew your food slowly. Saliva lubricates the food and predigests cooked starches. This signals your pancreas and small intestine to release the digestive enzymes and minerals they need to for digestion. Chewing also improves memory and reduces the release of stress hormones. Chewing also prevents food from putrefying and fermenting and prevents Candida overgrowth.

But chewing is more than a physical act. Try 'mindful' eating. Be conscious and fully aware of what you are eating as well as the act of eating. Make active choices while choosing the foods you eat, taking the time to look at your plate and notice the color, taste and texture of the food. Feelings of anger, tension and bickering and even chatting at meal times is stressful and disrupts digestion.

How does this assist weight loss? Studies have linked weight gain to chronic stress and you cannot get closer to linking weight gain to stress than at meal times!

▶ Keeping your body **hydrated** is another key to weight loss. Drink six to eight glasses of water every day. Pure, fresh water is best.

FOOD FACTS

Animal Proteins: What's the Beef?

The diet of a most Americans consists of meat and dairy products - steak, beef, mince pies, chicken and super-sized juicy hamburgers. Sure it's tasty, a taste the meat and poultry industry taught us to acquire. Did you know that Western societies consume at least 50 percent more protein than they actually need?

By filling up the connective tissues in our bodies with unused protein, we turn our bodies into overflowing pools of harmful acids and waste, thereby laying a fertile ground for disease. It also congests the digestive tract and overburdens the lymphatic system.

The fact is that animal proteins, unlike plant proteins, are difficult to digest. The human body is not able to adequately break down meat protein into amino acids. A healthy digestive system is in fact able to metabolize only 25 percent of the animal protein it ingests.

Chunks of undigested meat may therefore remain in the small intestine for as long as 20–48 hours, where they literally begin to rot. This generates the meat poisons, cadaverine, putrescine, amines and other highly toxic substances, which apart from causing disease also contributes to lymph congestion, fluid and fat build-up, first in the mid-section of the body, and eventually throughout the body.

The remnants of undigested meat can accumulate in the large intestinal for as long as - hold your breath – 20 to30 years or longer. Rotting meat also burdens the kidneys in the form of nitrogenous wastes. Even moderate meat-eaters demand three times more work from their kidneys than vegetarians do.

Here is something else to think about. Putrefaction and bacterial growth start immediately after an animal is slaughtered and are very advanced by the time the meat reaches most grocery stores or meat markets.

Destructive enzymes immediately begin to break down the cells in the cadaver's flesh, which leads to the formation of a degenerative substance called ptomaine that causes diseases.

Meat is also acid-forming and creates even more acidity when undigested. This, in turn, leads to a loss of minerals and other nutrients. Contrast this with plant proteins that the human body was designed to ingest in the course of evolution.

It is but a misconception that unlike meat, vegetables do not provide you with complete proteins - all the nine essential amino acids - that the body is unable to produce.

If you eat a variety of vegetables, you can get exactly the same amino acids as you get from meat - with added health benefits such as minerals and fiber that meat does not contain.

Vegetables: Pump Up the Volume

Not only are fruits and vegetables healthy, they can also directly assist with weight loss. Vegetables are high-volume foods i.e. they make you 'feel full' quicker than meat, poultry and dairy products do. That is why a vegetarian diet makes you eat less (and not because vegetables are less tasty than meat!). What's more, they are not high in calories. Hence, the weight-loss benefit.

Vegetables and fruits are also packed with nutrients that meat cannot give you, thereby not starving the body of certain types of nutrients. This explains why vegetarians, who eat a more well-rounded diet than meat-eaters, do not suffer food cravings.

Vegetables contain vitamins, minerals, enzymes, fiber, antioxidants and protein needed for good health and avoidance of disease.

According to research, the average American diet consists of only 8 percent fruits and vegetables. The problem is that the remaining 92 percent of the diet consists of nutritionally empty processed foods, low-carb and low-fat notwithstanding. This only fuels food cravings.

Also, you do not have to turn vegetarian to lose weight. Fruits and vegetables need to form the bulk of your diet, with meat and poultry eaten in small amounts and not necessarily with every meal.

Vegetables are also a good source of antioxidants, which counteract harmful 'free radicals'. These are unstable molecules which enter our bodies from various toxic sources. Some are even produced by the body itself.

Free radicals feed off healthy molecules to survive and if allowed free rein, they can cause cell damage that can lead to chronic and degenerative diseases.

The Fat's *Not* In The Fire!

We have been conditioned to believe that fat is Enemy Number One, especially for individuals who are overweight and obese. We have the low-fat craze of the 1980s and 1990s to thank for this message, so liberally fuelled by an overzealous media and a flood of weight-loss programs.

On the contrary, depriving your body of fats can lead to nutritional deficiencies and chronic disease. That is because fats are necessary for the absorption of nutrients from the food we eat. Many nutrients such as minerals, Beta carotene, Vitamin D, and Vitamin E are fat-soluble and can be metabolized and absorbed by the body only if there is sufficient fat in the diet.

The important thing is to choose healthy fats and to ingest them in moderate quantities. Healthy fats include extra-virgin olive oil, flax seed oil, and fats from plant sources such as nuts, seeds, avocados, and coconuts.

Fiber: All That Gas

We have been brainwashed with another mistaken notion - that large amounts of whole grain and bran-enriched foods aid digestion and elimination. We have also been told that bran-enriched breakfast cereals will make you eat less at lunch time.

While this is partially true, what is also true is that bran may actually be harmful to health. A high-fiber cereal for breakfast subdues Agni, which may make you eat less for lunch but makes you ravenous by dinner time!

However, in the evening, our digestive processes are subdued and this is not a good time to eat a hearty meal. An undigested meal will eventually result in the accumulation of toxic fecal matter in the intestines and you could *put on* weight despite all the bran you eat.

And this is only one of the ill-effects of whole-grain fiber. When all that bran enters your large intestine, it is attacked and broken down by bacteria that make it ferment and cause flatulence, headaches, irritability, fatigue, and sleep problems.

Also, food absorption through the gut wall should neither be slowed nor rushed. However, fiber abnormally speeds up food transportation through the gut, which leads to decreased nutrient absorption.

Eating fiber-enriched foods or foods containing rough fiber can significantly inhibit the absorption of iron, calcium, phosphorus, magnesium, sugars, proteins, fats and vitamins A, D, E and K. Phytates found in cereal fiber or bran, for instance, bind with calcium, iron and zinc making them indigestible, which in turn causes poor absorption.

Yes, fiber is essential for the elimination of waste from the bowel but make that *plant* fiber, not bran. Vegetable fiber does not putrefy in the intestine like bran does. It also makes for soft, large stools that are easy to eliminate. Bran, on the other hand, leads to the formation of small feces, which could get lodged in the folds of the colon.

Try to get your fiber from fresh fruit, salads, cooked grains, beans and vegetables. Cooked vegetables in particular contain plenty of fiber, which helps the digestive process but does not overwhelm the colon in the same way as bran does.

Also, the high water content of fruits and vegetables makes the passage through the intestinal tract much easier.

Salt: Gift from the Sea

Just like fats, salt is another much-maligned edible ingredient. We have been conditioned to believe that high sodium intake causes hypertension, arterial disease, kidney problems and water retention.

Yet imagine cooking without salt, or scrambled eggs without a sprinkling of salt. But more than these dishes, it is the salt in processed foods that causes disease and weight gain. Processed foods, apart from being nutritionally empty and causing abnormal spikes in blood sugar, contain generous quantities of salt and other sodium compounds. That is what sends your sodium levels shooting up.

So where's the catch? Our bodies need sodium to aid the absorption of major nutrients, for our nerves and muscles to function and to balance water and minerals in the internal environment. So salt is unavoidable, right?

Table salt, that ubiquitous condiment that most of us cannot do without, is highly refined, bleached and stripped of its minerals. Refined salt is actually more than 90 percent sodium, whereas unrefined, organic salt contains only 50 percent sodium. The rest is minerals and trace elements.

Some of the minerals present in unrefined salt that are absolutely essential to your body's healthy functioning are magnesium (an essential metabolic agent), calcium, potassium, and sulfate.

Contrast this with toxic chemicals such as aluminum, ferro cyanide, bleach and chlorine in refined salt and the difference to your health is evident.

pH Level: A Juggling Class Act

The human body performs many balancing acts, one of the most delicate being the acid-alkaline ratio. Obesity is a condition characterized by high toxicity levels, which make the blood and tissues acidic.

This could result from high levels of stress, a diet that tilts towards processed foods, meats and dairy products, and insufficient water intake. The body also produces its own acids such as hydrochloric acid for metabolism, bacteria and enzymes that release acids into the blood and tissues.

For the body to function at optimum capacity, it needs to be more alkaline than acid. This ratio is expressed as the pH balance (pH stands for 'power of hydrogen' or 'potential of hydrogen'). It is essentially the concentration of hydrogen ions in your blood and tissues. A body that has a blood pH of 7.4 is healthy. If the level falls below pH 7.34, you risk suffering from acidosis.

When acid levels climb, the body automatically leaches minerals from wherever they are available - calcium from bones and teeth - to neutralize the acids. The blood then dumps the acid into your organs and tissues, which then pour the acid back into the blood.

As part of your new and healthy weight-loss plan, minimize processed foods and meat in your diet, drink at least six to eight glasses of water every day, make sure you get some exercise, and work towards bringing down stress levels.

Medicating Yourself to Weight Gain?

You may think you are doing everything right but are still mysteriously putting on extra pounds. Weight gain is a complex issue and is linked to a number of factors. One of these is the medication you might be taking.

Some prescription drugs can actually cause you to put on weight, ranging from a few pounds to several pounds per month. Among the main culprits are steroids, anti-depressants, anti-psychotics, anti-seizure medications, birth-control pills, diabetes medications, and drugs to treat hypertension and heartburn.

These medical formulations act on different systems of the body, from appetite to insulin levels to fat storage to water retention.

Mid-Life Crisis

Weight gain may be a side-effect associated with certain medical conditions such as hypothyroidism, menopause, fibromyalgia, polycystic ovary syndrome and Cushing's Syndrome.

Hypothyroidism is a condition involving a deficiency of the thyroid hormones. The thyroid is directly linked to appetite control and responds to levels of the hormones leptin and ghrelin (See Chapter 11: Hour of Reckoning).

A deficiency in thyroid hormones causes metabolic disturbances that lower appetite and encourage fat storage and fluid retention, and consequent weight gain.

Many women also notice that menopause is accompanied by weight gain around the abdomen or mid-section. This is a process set off by fluctuating levels of the female hormone estrogen before and during menopause, and a lowering of estrogen after menopause.

Estrogen is produced mainly in the ovaries and contributes to the body's overall hormonal balance. Diminished estrogen levels make your body instinctively look for alternative sources of estrogen, such as adipose tissue and the skin. Since your fat cells are now helping you perform a critical balancing act, your body struggles to *keep* the adipose tissue and even thwarts weight-reduction efforts.

Also, estrogen along with adipose tissue is part of a complex biofeedback network that controls appetite, metabolism, digestion and detoxification. Throw any of these off-track and it leads to potential weight gain.

Worse still, if your diet is rich in processed foods and sugary drinks, and if you are subjected to chronic stress, you are likely to be insulin resistant. This makes you a prime candidate for weight gain.

Sleep Away The Pounds?

Surprising as this may sound, sleep loss or insufficient sleep could make you prone to putting on weight. In Chapter 11: Hour of Reckoning, I have discussed how imbalances in your sleeping pattern cause imbalances in the level of leptin, a hormone produced by fat cells, and another hormone, ghrelin, which is also linked to your appetite.

For a good night's rest, sleep before 10 pm, which also keeps melatonin levels normal (abnormal melatonin levels suppress thyroid hormones and thus can cause hypothyroidism and low metabolism, leading to weight gain).

Apart from late and erratic sleeping patterns, a condition called sleep apnea could also be adding to your weight. Prevalent more in middle-aged, overweight men than women, sleep apnea is a condition where you literally stop breathing periodically while asleep. These pauses in breathing could last for 5 to 10 seconds during each episode.

This disruptive sleep pattern, once again, affects levels of leptin and ghrelin, something that has been substantiated by numerous studies.

Exercise: Activate Your Life Force

Exercise is more than a state of physical activity. It energizes the life force, improves metabolism, increases immunity and releases 'happiness' hormones. And, yes, it also burns fat.

Over-exercising by engaging in aerobics, rigorous weight training and strenuous workouts harm the body (See Chapter 12: Energize, Not Exercise). So remain tuned to your body's capacity and body type, and choose the kind of exercise that is both comfortable and appropriate for you.

Here are some quick tips on how to energize yourself:

▶ A gentle, morning and/or evening walk is recommended

▶ Surya Namaskara or Sun Salutation is an ancient, complete and simple exercise program (as illustrated in Timeless *Secrets of Health and Rejuvenation*, or search the Internet for instructions; also See Chapter 12). It is a series of 12 postures repeated through two cycles and is a good all-round healer because it uses almost all the muscles in your body.

It improves respiration of all the body's cells, it Increases the chi or life force through important meridians, it pumps fluids and helps remove waste while delivering nutrients to your body's cells, it tones your hormonal system, and it also encourages regular bowel movements.

Start with just two cycles and gradually increase the number to eight or ten. Your body will start relying on chi, or the life force, for its energy requirements instead of using up its physical energy resources.

▶ Whenever you exercise, inhale through your nose while keeping your mouth closed to avoid harmful 'adrenaline breathing'. Mouth breathing rapidly depletes energy reserves and triggers the release of stress hormones.

▶ Exercise only up to 50 percent of your capacity.

▶ Expose your body to fresh air at least once or twice a day for at least half an hour each time.

▶ Regular practice of Yoga, Tai Chi, Chi Kung, Pilates or similar fitness programs is highly recommended for maintaining energy and flexibility.

▶ Pranayama: Five-minute breathing exercises to increase Prana or Chi. This is best done before meditation and before eating.

▶ Meditation according to your choice: I recommend the 'Technique of Conscious Breathing' as described in my book *It's Time to Come Alive.*

Sunny Side Up!

Complementing your exercise program with regular exposure to sunlight is the perfect way to activate the life force within you. It is not difficult to conclude that morning is the best time to exercise - outdoors.

Whether it is a morning walk, jog, PACE interval training or Surya Namaskara (See Chapter 12: Energize, Not Exercise), getting out there and energizing your chi will keep you invigorated for the rest of the day.

Regular sun exposure has seemingly endless benefits. Studies reveal that exposing patients to controlled amounts of sunlight dramatically lowers elevated blood pressure (up to 40 mm Hg drop), decreases cholesterol in the bloodstream, lowers abnormally high blood sugar in diabetics, and increases the number of white blood cells which you need to resist disease.

The ultraviolet band of sunlight also activates a skin hormone called solitrol. Solitrol influences our immune system and many of our body's regulatory centers, and, in conjunction with the pineal hormone melatonin, causes changes in mood and daily biological rhythms.

The hemoglobin in our red blood cells requires ultraviolet light to bind to the oxygen needed for all cellular functions. Lack of sunlight can, therefore, be held co-responsible for almost any kind of illness.

Sunlight also stimulates Vitamin D, which is actually a group of vitamins that play an important part in bone growth and development, and in the absorption of minerals by the blood. Vitamin D deficiency can lead to a wide variety of diseases.

Soaking in as little as 15 minutes of the mid-day sun is enough for the body to manufacture all the Vitamin D it needs.

Individuals who live in the Northern latitudes, where the sun is weak and winters are long, may use a 'Vitamin D lamp' (or UV lamp).

While sunlight and Vitamin D may not seem to have a direct bearing on weight loss, it is a vital component while re-balancing the new and healthy lifestyle you have embraced as part of your overall weight-reduction and health plan.

Obesity Is a State of Mind

What would you say if I told you that obesity is a state of mind? Let me put it this way. Obesity has as much to do with storing fat as it has to do with your perceptions of yourself and the world around you.

It is a vital link - perhaps *the* most vital link - that conventional medicine missed. Lots of people live toxic lifestyles, not only individuals who are obese, it's just that different bodies adjust and react to toxicity in different ways. Individuals who are obese tend to store physical as well as emotional toxins in their fat cells.

What you think, how you perceive yourself and others, and the basic assumptions and premises by which you live have a profound effect on your weight. I have elaborated on the subject earlier (See Chapter 4: The Big Three), where I have discussed destructive thought patterns, carrying the baggage of emotional traumas, the stress response, and one's negative beliefs about being overweight.

For any type of real physical, mental or spiritual healing to take place, you must make an important decision, perhaps one of the most important you will ever make. Depending on which way you look at it, it could also be one of the easiest or one of the most difficult decisions you will ever make. It is a decision to become emotionally whole, or simply, a decision to heal yourself.

It is a demonstrated fact that techniques of physical, mental, and spiritual healing cause physiological changes in the brain and other organs. That is because our thoughts, beliefs and emotions are stored not only in our cerebral cortex but also in our cells and tissues via complex neural pathways powered by chemical messengers called neurotransmitters.

Though natural healing techniques impact on this cellular memory, remember that this journey starts in mind - with a decision you have made to heal yourself, to clearly see the mind-body connection at work and to rely on your innate wisdom to cure yourself.

If you would prefer to start with baby steps, begin by creating the time and space to access your healing force. Simply spend some quiet time by yourself every day, perhaps in the park or even sit up in bed when you wake up every morning and before you sleep every night and 'empty' your mind.

Repeat this for a few days and you will already begin to feel the difference! Detoxifying you mind in this way will instantly relieve stress. This will, in turn, start the positive loop you need to take the power of internal healing even further.

Different things work for different people. So find your own stress-busters, such as a walk around the block after your evening meal, playing with your pet, watching the sunset or even sitting with your feet up and doing absolutely nothing.

Once you begin to experience the benefits of these simple practices, you will embrace an attitude of relaxation rather than the stress-filled life so many people are almost addicted to. You might then want to explore other systems that re-balance and unite the mind and body such as progressive relaxation, deep breathing, meditation, and yoga.

Remember, being overweight is indeed a state of mind.

Chapter 11: Hour of Reckoning

Get Some R&R: Rest & Repair

Sleep, like everything else in the human body, follows nature's biological clock. This is called the circadian rhythm, and it controls every aspect of the body, its organs, tissues, hormones and functions such as digestion, elimination and renewal.

Sleep is the resting stage of the body and is required so that our tissues and organs can repair and recharge themselves. According to nature's clock, the body begins to switch off and wind down in the late evening, which is when the processes of purification and renewal begin to take over.

What exactly takes place during this nocturnal hour? For instance, growth hormones, responsible for cellular growth, repair and rejuvenation, are secreted profusely between 10 pm and midnight. Between midnight and 2 am, the liver receives most of the body's energy to conduct as many as 500-odd different functions.

Since we are not consciously aware of these processes, we often do not realize how important it is to synchronize our sleep patterns with the body's natural rhythms.

The body's level of activity, sleep and alertness is regulated by two hormones - serotonin and melatonin - both of which are secreted in tandem with the circadian rhythm. Since the circadian rhythm follows the movements of the sun, it is important to sleep at the appropriate time (10 pm) and wake up at sunrise (usually 6 am).

Though it may seem farfetched at first, weight gain and obesity is not only a factor of what we eat but how much sleep we get and when we turn in for the night as well.

Extensive research has been conducted in this area, consistently connecting chronic sleep deprivation - turning in too late, keeping up all night, disturbed sleep, and erratic sleeping habits - to higher body mass and obesity in adults as well as in children. In fact, researchers have found that the younger the individual, the more intimate the connection.

Research also suggests that sleep deprivation is linked to glucose intolerance and insulin resistance of the kind seen in type 2 diabetes.

Over the last three to four decades, more and more Americans have been sleeping for shorter durations at bedtime. This has become a feature of modern society, with both children and adults having shorter bedtimes than, say, 30 years ago.

This trend coincides with the period during which there has been a dramatic increase in the prevalence of obesity in the US. During the same period, studies have found an increase in obesity among American children and teenagers, aged 2–5, 6–11, and 12–19, from the early '70s. In each age group, the prevalence of obesity tripled over the last three decades.

Is this pure coincidence or is there a closer relationship between sleep deprivation and being overweight? Research, from both long-term studies as well as in laboratory settings, indicates that chronic partial sleep loss, in other words, shorter bedtimes, may increase the risk of weight gain and obesity.

This is possibly due to a constellation of factors such as metabolic and endocrine alterations, including decreased glucose tolerance, decreased insulin sensitivity, elevated evening concentrations of cortisol, increased levels of ghrelin, decreased levels of leptin, and increased hunger and appetite.

Simply put, sleep plays a significant role in the regulation of the body's neuroendocrine functions and glucose metabolism in children as well as in adults. This means sleep is intrinsically linked to the body's hormonal functions as well as its metabolism or energy homeostasis.

Partial sleep deprivation or over a prolonged period, as witnessed in modern lifestyles, can cause long-lasting biochemical changes that disturb the delicate balance between the hormones that regulate appetite and metabolism.

These changes are believed to eventually lead to increased appetite and overeating, weight gain and obesity.

The key facts here are two hormones - leptin and ghrelin. Loosely understood, while leptin suppresses appetite, ghrelin stimulates it. Let us take a look at each one separately, and the roles they play in hunger and appetite.

Leptin: Midnight Hunger

Leptin is a protein hormone produced by the body's adipose tissue, or simply, fat cells. Yes, adipose tissue or body fat - apart from storing energy and cushioning and insulating the body - is also an endocrine organ that synthesizes many protein hormones.

Interestingly, the realization that adipose tissue was an endocrine organ is, in fact, attributed to the discovery of leptin in 1994.

Leptin lets your brain know when your body has eaten enough food. High levels of leptin then signal satiety and prompt the individual to stop eating. Alternatively, low levels of leptin signal hunger and lead to increased food intake.

This hormone works the other way around too, to regulate energy balance. When you are deprived of food and therefore lack sufficient energy, leptin levels fall significantly. This signals the brain to make you feel hungry so that your body replenishes its energy through immediate food intake.

Alternatively, when energy levels are optimal, leptin levels rise. This hormone signals the brain that the body is satiated and suppresses appetite. The result: you are likely to say no to a second helping at dinner.

In laboratory settings, it has been observed that leptin is more sensitive to starvation than overfeeding i.e. leptin levels fall significantly during starvation but do not rise significantly due to overeating.

Studies indicate that leptin is also highly sensitive to the amount of sleep you get. One such study found that mean leptin levels were as much as 19 percent lower when subjects were allowed four hours of sleep compared to subjects who had twelve hours of sleep.

This seems to explain why some individuals who turn in to bed at night but find it difficult to sleep can rest easy only after a midnight snack!

Though the rules by which the human body works apply to everyone, individual differences and differences in biochemistry have made for certain unique findings in research. Some studies have found that the brain can become resistant to leptin, adding another dimension to the sleep-obesity link.

Research has also found that some obese individuals have high levels of leptin circulating in their blood but are resistant to its effects, leading to overeating.

Ghrelin: Growing Appetite

Leptin is only half the side of the sleep-obesity story. The other half is determined by another hormone called ghrelin.

Ghrelin is identified primarily as a growth hormone that also plays an important role in hunger, appetite and energy regulation. Discovered in 1999, five years after leptin was discovered, ghrelin is also important to learning and memory.

This hormone is produced mainly in the stomach and pancreas as well as in the hypothalamus. High levels of ghrelin stimulate hunger.

When the body's energy reserves are depleted, ghrelin makes the body store fat to conserve energy. It also decreases the breakdown of fat stores so that energy is not further depleted.

Ghrelin appears to act independently of leptin. Sleep deprivation is associated with increased levels of ghrelin and increased appetite. Research shows that sleep-deprived subjects, particularly, have a strong appetite for high-carbohydrate foods. That is why many processed foods are perhaps preferred midnight snacks!

Sleep deprivation is also associated with a nearly 40 percent decrease in glucose tolerance. This reduction in glucose tolerance is associated with decreased insulin sensitivity.

The combination of these two metabolic deficiencies indicates an increased risk of type 2 diabetes. Reduced insulin sensitivity is also associated with an increased risk of obesity, often referred to a companion disease to diabetes.

Despite the considerable research on ghrelin, scientists are still not sure of the exact nature of the relationship between levels of this hormone and obesity.

Hormones act in complex ways, and to suggest any cause-and-effect link between either leptin or ghrelin, and obesity would be premature. But what is certain is that there *is* a link between these hormones and weight gain.

Paying For Sleep Debt

According to some estimates, Americans average about six hours of sleep per night. That may be enough for some, but not for the majority of people, especially for those concerned about their weight.

A study from Columbia University, presented at the annual scientific meeting of the North American Association for the Study of Obesity, found that people need to get a lot more than six hours of sleep each night to stay healthy and fit.

Researchers used almost 10 years of data collected on nearly 18,000 subjects who took part in the National Health and Nutrition Examination Survey (NHANES). The study gathered information on general dietary and health habits. After accounting for other factors known to contribute to obesity, the Columbia team reported these findings:

- Less than 4 hours of sleep per night increases the obesity risk by 73 percent compared to subjects who slept 7 to 9 hours each night
- An average 5 hours of sleep per night increases obesity risk by 50 percent
- An average 6 hours of sleep per night increases obesity risk by 23 percent

Researchers with the Departments of Medicine and Health Studies, University of Chicago, cited the following findings in a paper presented in 2008. The paper quotes a survey conducted by the American Cancer Society in 1960 that found average sleep duration to be 8 to 8.9 hours in the general population. That was then.

Thirty-five years later, a survey conducted by the National Sleep Foundation in 1995, found that average sleep duration had dropped to seven hours. Today, more than 30 percent of adult men and women aged between 30 and 64 get less than 6 hours of sleep every night.

The same general consequences of sleep curtailment apply to children. A November 2007 National Institute of Child Health and Human Development Study of Early Child Care and Youth Development found that overweight sixth-graders slept less than children who were not overweight.

The study also showed that for every additional hour of sleep in the third grade, a child was 40 percent less likely to be overweight in the sixth grade.

Research on sleep patterns and obesity also reveal that younger children seem to need at least 9 hours of sleep, whereas teenagers actually need 10 to 12 hours of sleep to remain slim and healthy.

Tune In to Your Body Clock

To understand just why this is supremely important, let us return to the biological rhythms mentioned earlier in this chapter. Why is it so very important to sleep at a specific time every night? And why is it important to maintain this cycle? What happens when the body is not in sync with these rhythms?

Imagine each bodily process as being controlled by a biological timer. Then think of each timer being hooked to a master clock.

The master clock coordinates all the individual clocks with each other and makes certain that every activity in the body is carried out according to its master plan. This master plan consists of nothing but the body's constant effort to maintain perfect equilibrium or balance.

The body's master clock is controlled by nature's most influential cycle called the circadian rhythm. The circadian rhythm makes us wake up in the morning, makes us most active in the morning and causes us to wind down in the evening.

We also mentioned two important hormones earlier - melatonin and serotonin - which are intrinsically linked to our daily sleep and wakefulness rhythms. The secretion of melatonin follows a regular 24-hour rhythm. Melatonin production reaches peak levels between 1 am and 3 am, and drops to its lowest levels at midday.

Since the pineal gland, which secretes this hormone, releases it directly into the bloodstream, it is instantly made available to every cell in the body and tells them 'what time it is'.

The brain synthesizes another important hormone called serotonin. This hormone has a powerful influence on day and night rhythms, sexual behavior, memory, appetite, impulsiveness, fear and even suicidal tendencies.

Unlike melatonin, serotonin increases with the light of day, with peak secretions at midday, and also through physical exercise and the intake of sugar.

Having understood just why it is important to have regularity in one's life, let us take a look at modern lifestyles.

The rhythm of life has changed dramatically in urban society in the developed world over the last three decades. This fast-paced life has brought many wonderful changes in the form of night life, cable and satellite TV, night shifts, an increase in travel across time zones, and the invention of the microchip, all of which has us in always-on mode.

As we made the shift from a simpler, more predictable way of life to a 24x7, seven-days-a-week lifestyle, we have become unmindful of the effects on our health. Sleep was one of the first things to take the fall.

Add to this the invention of fast food and its aggressive promotion by monopolistic corporations that literally feed off the empty calories they dump into your body and you have a recipe for obesity.

The National Center for Health Statistics went door-to-door and interviewed more than 87,000 adults between 2004 and 2006. The center's findings suggested a definite connection between sleep loss and obesity.

One third of the people who slept less than 6 hours were obese, while only 22 percent of those who slept for 7 to 8 hours were obese.

If you are trying to lose weight, getting enough sleep should be on your list of priorities. Getting the right amount of sleep would make sure you restore your ghrelin-leptin balance to naturally maintain your optimal weight.

You must also make sure you sleep at the right time. Sleeping excessively late or not sleeping at all and trying to make up for it with too much sleep only confuses your body and throws the leptin-ghrelin equilibrium out of gear.

Thumb rule: Flip your biological switch and turn off the lights at around 10 pm. Then try to get at least 8 hours of sleep every night. If you surrender to nature's rhythm, your body will gladly respond with weight loss and a basket of other health benefits.

Chapter 12: Energize, Not Exercise

Why Exercise?

If you are overweight, chances are that 'diet' and 'exercise' are the two most oft-repeated words you have spoken or heard.

They are also top of the vocabulary for dieticians, nutritionists and weight-loss 'experts', who believe in using simple formulae to help people lose weight.

The problem with this approach is that it takes a symptomatic view of the human body and says: "Cut the calories and burn the fat" and you are sure to lose weight.

What invariably follows is an array of complex food charts, a regimen of strenuous exercise (often a different set for a different body part) and a weighing scale to measure the success or failure of your weight-loss plan.

Approaches such as these use two principles which, according to me, are fundamentally flawed. According to them, the symptom (obesity) is the disease, and the body the sum of its parts.

These experts then use a whole jargon of complex words to explain simple biological processes. Sometimes, one tends to think this is a deliberate attempt to keep the public in the dark!

Ignorance breeds insecurity and fear, leaving people with no option other than to turn to these medical 'experts' for an effective 'cure', in this case, weight-loss 'experts'.

What if I were to tell you that weight loss can be a painless process? And that it does not involve an exhausting exercise routine? But before we get to that, let us take a look at why exercise is one of the fundaments of weight loss and good health.

Switch now from viewing your body as a human machine that merely ingests food and then burns it as fuel or stores it as unwanted fat. Set aside diet and exercise and exercise formulae, for a moment, and think of your body as a dynamic, living being with energy in constant motion.

To function optimally - and to maintain ideal body weight - every bodily process must be carried out as nature intended. For this to take place, your energy needs to flow in a certain way. Most of all, it needs to be in balance and also in harmony with your environment and the universe. But how is this possible? How does a body that is way off-track return to a state of equilibrium?

Nature never intended for us to live the sedentary lives many of us lead thanks to advancements in technology that have replaced natural daily activities. Neither were we meant to virtually career from one situation to another, traveling the way many of us do, craving entertainment, multi-tasking and bombarding our senses with electronic stimulation.

The human body requires an adequate amount of daily activity to keep its energies in motion. This dynamically powers every physiological and biochemical process that keeps us alive and in a state of good health and well-being.

For instance, it enhances our capacity to digest food, metabolize it, and eliminate physical and emotional impurities. It keeps our body firm and supple, and increases our ability to deal with stress.

It also keeps the lymphatic system, which accounts for most of our immune system, functioning at optimal capacity. Unlike blood, which has the heart to keep it circulating, the lymph literally depends on physical activity to stay fine-tuned.

The lymphatic system, in fact, relies heavily on our breathing mechanism, which with the help of the diaphragm, forces the lymph to move through the lymph ducts and vessels. Hence, in addition to building lung capacity and purifying the blood, gentle breathing exercises enhance our immune system and help us de-stress.

Alternatively, shallow breathing, which results from a sedentary lifestyle, impairs proper lymph drainage.

A brisk walk, a gentle jog and cycling, for instance, all enhance breathing as do mind-body exercises and meditation techniques such as yoga.

Here is an interesting finding: According to a research study, published in August 2009, practicing yoga can significantly reduce the risk of being obese. The study, conducted by the Fred Hutchinson Cancer Research Center and published in the *Journal of the American Dietetic Association,* found that that this had more to do with what the researchers called 'mindful eating' than the physical aspect of yoga.

Yoga in general sensitizes the mind to various bodily processes and thereby creates a need for healthy living and practices. It also facilitates the crucial connect between mind and body that is woefully lacking in most individuals in Western society today.

According to the researchers, individuals who 'eat mindfully' are acutely aware of their appetite - both feelings of hunger as well as satiety. So they eat when hungry and stop when they are full. This takes place when one is aware of the signals the body sends out in response to food or the lack or excess of it.

Responding to the needs of 'real' appetite, as opposed to overeating or snacking mindlessly, controls intake and therefore keeps one's weight in check.

There is also a more subtle change that takes place in yoga practitioners - the need to live healthy translates into a need to also eat healthy. Which means one is naturally disinclined to eat chemically-laced processed foods and beverages that fill the body with chemical poisons.

This is corroborated by researchers at the Fred Hutchinson Cancer Research Center, who found that the 'mindful eating' meant the subjects in their study were aware of why they were eating and how the food they were eating was good for their health.

Interestingly, the researchers did not find any correlation between other types of physical activity such as walking or running, and mindful eating. Hence, they concluded that including yoga in any weight-loss program could make it more effective.

Physical exercise such as walking, running, jogging, swimming, in moderation is a great immune stimulant. It improves neuromuscular integration across age groups. As oxygen courses through our cells, we experience a sense of well-being. This in turn boosts self-confidence and self-esteem.

Don't Push It

Demanding workouts, with weights, for instance, trigger the stress response, which in turn leads to weight gain. That is because vigorous workouts cause the secretion of abnormal amounts of stress hormones such as adrenaline and cortisol.

Cortisol is released when the body needs a sudden surge of energy to deal with a threat or real and present danger. When this happens, the body musters energy from its reserves at short notice to supply more fuel fur immediate use.

Anthropologists who study human evolution call this the 'fight or flight' response, both instinctive reactions to a predatory threat that prompts an individual to either confront the threat or run away from it.

How does the body suddenly muster fuel at a second's notice? It secretes cortisol which draws on two energy sources - it quickly metabolizes proteins from the muscles and converts them into glycogen or blood sugar. It also draws on stored fat and burns it to supply the added fuel that may be needed.

The body perceives a grueling exercise routine as a threat because such workouts demand sudden energy. That is exactly how the brain interprets strenuous exercise.

This is counterproductive for three reasons. One, consistently high levels of blood glucose trigger insulin resistance and this in turn leads to weight gain.

The second reason why tiring workouts are unhealthy is that cortisol literally depletes or eats away at your muscles. Since the stress response draws on energy reserves, it drains away energy and leaves the body unable to repair the tissues and muscles. Once the adrenaline rush is over, the side-effects start kicking in.

But don't drastic weight-reduction plans produce dramatic results? What about all those people on television talk shows who lose, say, 20 pounds in 30 days or 100 pounds in 9 months?

Yes, but what is not quite so publicly publicized is that about half the overweight individuals who subject themselves to such physical 'abuse' regain their lost weight in 12 months. Those who don't, have to keep up the rigorous and punishing routines or risk putting it all back on.

Conventional weight-loss plans place a tremendous strain on the human body, prompting many to give up mid-way. Slacken the routine just a little and you gain the weight you lost by starving and sweating it out.

This can be devastating and many individuals give up trying altogether. The message you are sending their body is: "It is impossible for me to lose weight. I am always going to be overweight."

This brings us to the third detrimental consequence of strenuous workouts such as long sessions of aerobics or endurance training. Why do so many overweight individuals regain the weight they shed when they stop working out?

There is a fundamental flaw to exercising to the point of exhaustion - it burns fat, which is the wrong fuel! As shocking as that might sound, this is how it works at the physiological level. Extended workouts, or exercising for more than 20 minutes, releases cortisol, which in turn burns fat for fuel during the exercise session.

Since fat reserves are depleted, your body then synthesizes and stores more fat to replenish the depleted reserves in preparation for the next workout. With every successive workout, the fat-burning-fat storing cycle is further established till the body learns that it must make and store more fat every time some is burned.

Hence, long and punishing workouts actually make the body store fat. That doesn't seem to be a problem as long as you keep on exercising and burning the fat that builds up. Slow down a little and weight gain sets in.

PACE It Out

A healthy alternative is interval training. Going by the rather formidable term 'Progressively Accelerating Cardiopulmonary Exertion' or simple PACE, this means engaging in very short bursts of intense exercise followed by a very short period of rest and recovery.

Choose an exercise that suits you - like jogging, spot running, skipping or using an exercise bike. Engage in a short, intense burst of exercise lasting for no more than 30 seconds, then stop and rest for two minutes. Repeat this four times and you're done exercising for the day - in eight minutes flat!

Now repeat this three to four times a week and not only will you lose weight, you will feel revitalized, rejuvenated and invigorated with an enhanced cardiovascular capacity, and lean and strong muscles, among many other health benefits.

How does interval training or PACE work at the physiological level? Why doesn't it cause the same devastating effects as aerobic exercise?

When you exercise in short bursts, your body burns carbohydrates in the form of stored glycogen stored in the muscles and liver. It doesn't burn fat during the session. After each session, it starts burning fat to replenish the depleted glycogen from your muscles and liver which were used during your training session.

Your body then continues to metabolize and burn fat for the next 24 hours after your interval training session. Your body thus learns that it does not have to store fat only to burn it again during a rigorous workout but that it must slowly burn fat to replenish depleted glycogen reserves. This is called afterburn, a magical and automatic process you can in motion by simply tweaking the type of exercise!

And in case it didn't strike you - do the math and you'll realize you need to exercise for quite literally less than 10 minutes a day! How's that for people who are pressed for time?

The medical journal, *Lancet*, reports that aerobic exercise can cause deadly arterial clogging and heart disease in those who had never before had heart trouble. According to *The American Journal of Cardiology*, jogging has similarly caused some runners to drop dead from heart attacks. Their autopsies show severe coronary artery disease. Any regular, strenuous form of exercise actually does about as much damage to your heart as continuous stress does.

The heart literally comes under constant attack via the excessive exercise sessions. Marathon runners are known to lose muscle mass, both in the heart and the rest of the body. Many have dropped dead just after reaching the finishing line.

Three people died during the Boston Marathon in 2009 - aged 26, 36 and 65. That is not all. In 2008, a young woman died three miles before the finish line during the Dallas White Rock Marathon.

In 2007, two high-profile marathon deaths were reported, one in Chicago and the other during the Olympic trials in New York. In the UK that year, another runner collapsed and died during the London Marathon. In 2006, at least six participants died in various marathons in the US.

The sponsors of these events and even some doctors call these deaths a 'statistical fluke'. However, research suggests otherwise. Studies conducted by hospitals in Boston on marathon runners over the last decade reveals that marathon-running *increases* cardiac risk.

These studies showed that men and women marathon runners in fact increased the risk of cardiac arrest, sudden cardiac death, and developing hardened arteries, lower back pain, repetitive stress injuries, stress fractures, blood in the urine and permanent bone damage.

Dr Arthur Siegel, director of Internal Medicine at McLean Hospital in Massachusetts and an Assistant Professor of Medicine at Harvard University, has extensively studied the effects of the Boston Marathon.

Dr Arthur Siegel has found that participants showed cardiac damage similar to the symptoms that appear during a heart attack 24 hours after the race.

This happens because, over a period of time, the body adapts to marathon-like conditions. It therefore reduces the capacity of the heart and lungs to conserve energy so that it can go the extra mile. In other words, it begins to economize on a daily basis. Marathon training therefore actually trains the heart to get weaker.

Vigorous weight training is also self-defeating. It leads to abnormally enlarged, bloated muscle fibers that actually become dysfunctional and prone to injuries. Oversized muscles constantly use up a lot of precious energy (complex sugar reserves), energy that your body requires for its more important activities.

Weight training also adds excessive muscle tissue to parts of the body where it was never designed to be, thus hindering natural patterns of movement. Lifting heavy weights can also raise your blood pressure and increase the risk of strokes and aneurysms.

By nature, the human body was not made to deal with the additional gravitational force imposed on it while lifting heavy weights. Frequently stressing the joints, muscles and tendons causes them to age prematurely.

Let us briefly look at what happens when the body is pushed to the limits of endurance and then beyond. It is a phenomenon experienced by marathon runners. Why is it addictive and why is endurance running not recommended?

Marathon and cross-country training gives athletes a 'runner's high'. When you push your body beyond its threshold of endurance, the pituitary gland begins to secrete a neurotransmitter called endorphins. These endorphins suppress pain and allow the body to be pushed even further, an evolutionary response when man had to hunt and forage in harsh terrain.

This is precisely what happens to players of aggressive competitive sports such as wrestling, weight-lifting, rugby and ice hockey. Players keep going despite bloody wounds, unmindful of bodily injury.

The most effective type of physical exercise is that which mirrors evolutionary patterns - hunting and foraging involved short and intense bursts of energy.

Tips For Exercising

If interval training is the best form of exercise, that does not mean you shouldn't walk, jog or swim to energize your body if you would like to. Here are some useful tips that will help you get the most out of your exercise routine.

Exercise to only half your capacity. Tiring yourself only defeats the very purpose. Exercise is supposed to make you feel refreshed, revitalized and energetic. As you proceed, your capacity for exercise will naturally increase.

How do you know when to stop? That's easy. When you start breathing through your mouth rather than through your nose, it is a sign that your body is going into stress mode and is about to start drawing on reserves. You definitely don't want that. This is also called adrenaline-breathing mode. When this happens, taper off with a short period of walking and normal breathing. A good thumb rule is to exercise to the point of perspiration once a day.

We need strong muscles to meet the typical demands of the day. The best way to increase muscle tone and strength is to quickly raise heart and muscle activity to the point of panting, followed by a period of low activity (or 'active recovery'). One to two-minute intervals (of activity and rest) are ideal.

Doing this for 10–20 minutes a day is more beneficial than hours of strenuous exercise. It increases muscle tone, lung capacity and heart health.

During the panting phases, the body uses up its complex sugar reserves in the muscles. For those who desire weight loss, this method causes you to lose weight after exercising, as the body tries to replenish its lost sugar reserves by breaking down fat deposits while you are resting.

Weight loss achieved during strenuous endurance exercise programs, on the other hand, tends to be reversed because the body tries to quickly replenish the lost fat deposits to prepare itself for the next energy-depleting round of exercise. The body perceives the strenuous exercise as a threat.

Another thumb rule is to exercise during daylight hours. This is in keeping with the body's natural rhythms and when you go with the flow of energy, you get maximum benefit. The best time to exercise is between 6 am and 10 am, and late afternoon between 5 pm and 6 pm. 'Hitting the gym' after work, as so many people love to call it, is not a good idea. This is because the body begins to wind down after sunset.

Also, never exercise just before or after a meal as this impairs Agni the digestive fire, and leads to indigestion. However, taking a walk for 15 minutes after meals works as a good digestive aid. Another tip: always drink water before and after exercising to prevent the blood from thickening and the cells from becoming dehydrated.

Body Drought

It may appear farfetched at first but dehydration is often linked to being overweight. One reason why so many Americans are dehydrated is that beverages such as tea, coffee, colas and other soft drinks have become primary thirst-quenchers.

All these drinks are powerful diuretics or agents that stimulate urination. Caffeine in tea and coffee, for instance, is a nerve toxin that the body ties to remove as soon as it senses its presence in the blood.

The best and most efficient way to remove a poison from the blood is to mix it with water and excrete it via urination.

Yet the importance of drinking sufficient quantities of water - six to eight 8-ounce glasses a day - cannot be underestimated. The human body is 70 percent water, mirroring the percentage of water on the planet.

Every one of the 60–100 trillion cells in the body depends on this life-giving, purifying fluid so that the body can perform its myriad functions effectively.

To protect themselves against further loss of water, dehydrated cells make their membranes almost impermeable to water diffusion, while drawing in excess fats, including cholesterol.

This is only a survival mechanism but one that has devastating consequences over time. In severely dehydrated individuals, it prevents metabolic waste from leaving the cells, causing them to suffocate in their own waste. Sometimes, cells eventually mutate and turn cancerous to survive in this toxic environment.

Dehydration also causes a craving for salty foods, which is why fast foods like potato chips and popcorn are irresistible. These foods, as we know, are among the biggest culprits for weight gain and obesity.

But what causes these food cravings? It is the kidneys' way of making sure they get sufficient salt or sodium to hold on to the little water left in the body. This in turn compounds the effects of an already dehydrated body.

As the body holds on to more and more water or moisture ingested through food intake, the water accumulates in the fluid outside the cells. This is because the impermeable cell membranes fail to draw in the water they so badly need. This stagnating water leads to water retention and weight gain.

A body that has survived in a state of drought for years needs to be re-hydrated very gradually. Any sudden intake of large amounts of water can indeed cause severe lymph congestion, swelling, and in some cases, even death.

This is called 'water intoxication', a potentially fatal disturbance in brain function that occurs when the normal balance of electrolytes in the body is pushed outside safe limits by a rapid intake of water.

Sometimes, the transition from severe dehydration to re-hydration is best monitored by a health practitioner.

Both water and salt are absolutely essential for balanced water metabolism and to generate enough hydroelectric energy to maintain cellular activities. Drinking water and eliminating energy-depleting and overstimulating beverages are usually the first line of treatment in case of any illness. In some cases, all that is required is re-hydration and sufficient rest.

Life Energies

Health experts may not all agree on the most effective type of exercise and the amount you should get. But they are unanimous that just like the Big Four - heart disease, cancer, diabetes and obesity - have reached epidemic proportions in Western countries, physical inactivity is also looked upon as a disease of alarming proportions.

Besides, physical inactivity is also closely linked to the Big Four, perhaps more directly than most of us realize.

Just as the human body was not designed for prolonged and intense activity, it was also not meant to be inactive. It is simply not nature's way. It is the same principle on which your car battery works. If you don't charge it for a while, it malfunctions and then dies altogether (the ultimate state of inactivity).

The bottom line: recharging your energies regularly, or simply living a physically active life, is fundamental to keeping the body ticking. It is the basic life force that keeps every cell in your body alive and working.

The sedentary life that most people in Western societies live blocks the life force, locks it up in various organs and tissues and distorts it into a diseased state. Good health, or alternatively ill-health, depends on whether our habits and daily routines are in harmony with the life force and natural rhythms both inside our bodies and which connect us to the environment and the universe.

In simple words, partying when the body needs to be resting, exercising when it needs to focus on digestion, sleeping when the body's natural energies are at their peak or physical inactivity distort the body's energies and the processes they are responsible for.

So what exactly are these energies? The human constitution is composed of three doshas or dynamic forces of nature. The doshas are composed of the five basic elements that make up the universe - earth, water, fire, air and space.

These five elements are essentially energies that vibrate at different frequencies. For instance, the photons or particles of light that are constantly generated in the air that surrounds you, have a different pattern of energy than energy created by particles in a clump of clay or the water that flows in a river.

All existing matter, no matter how dense, is but a constant intermingling of these five elements or vibrational energies. In the body, these elemental energies are grouped together and represented as the three doshas - Pitta (predominantly fire with some water), Vata (both air and space) and Kapha (predominantly water with some earth).

Each dosha is responsible for a different set of physiological processes, each one is different from the other, each one performs different functions, and each one is more or less predominant at a different time of day or night.

The human body is in constant search for equilibrium. Thus, balancing the doshas and allowing them to perform their roles as they were naturally intended is the key to maintaining weight loss, longevity and good health.

It's all about gradually transforming your lifestyle from one that is highly toxic to one that is in harmony with your body's natural rhythms. I will briefly summarize each dosha because they relate to human body type, something that determines your optimal body weight.

Vata - 'Moving' Force: Vata translates as 'air' or movement, transporting food, air, water, blood, lymph and waste through the body. The nervous system, circulatory system, lymphatic system, digestive tract, bronchi and lungs, bile ducts, hormonal pathways, and cellular ducts are all part of an enormously complex network, sustained by the movement and power of Vata.

Excessive Vata results in hyperactivity and hypertension. If Vata slows down and comes to a halt, constipation or bile duct blockage may occur. Congestion of the coronary arteries, blood vessel walls, lymph nodes, urinary ducts, prostate gland, uterus, sinuses, thyroid gland and other areas of the body all result from disturbed Vata activity.

The blocked flow of Vata is responsible for the hundreds of diseases that conventional medicine tries to treat away with drugs or medication without giving due attention to what causes the congestion.

Vata's primary seat is the colon. If the large intestine is clear of obstructions, Vata is able to perform its important activities throughout the rest of the body. When disturbed, Vata problems leads to abdominal distention, gas and constipation, such accumulated Vata may result in obesity or what is called 'anabolic Vata'.

Pitta - Dynamic Energy: The small intestine is mainly controlled by the energy of Pitta - the second dosha. Pitta, which in Sanskrit means 'bile', controls Agni and, therefore, digestion and metabolism. Pitta ensures that food is properly digested, absorbed and metabolized.

Once the Pitta-dosha becomes disturbed at its main seat, where the gallbladder and pancreas are joined with the duodenum, all metabolic processes are disrupted. Consequently, the assimilation and metabolism of nutrients becomes insufficient, and the body suffers the effects of malnourishment, even if the person eats well. Being overweight indicates that the body has reached this stage of intestinal dysfunction.

If Vata continues to act in its reversed mode, intestinal toxins and waste fragments, as well as portions of the bile released by the gallbladder and enzymes released by the pancreas, are pushed further toward the stomach. A continued diminished availability of bile and digestive enzymes can lead to obesity, which is a condition of advanced cellular starvation, as well as to heart disease and cancer.

Kapha - Integration and Stamina: The third principal force that controls the human body is Kapha. This dosha stands for cohesion, structure, stamina and strength. Its main seat is in the stomach and chest. Kapha controls the digestive juices and forms the connective tissue (the interstitial fluid surrounding cells), muscles, fat, bones and sinew.

It also lubricates the joints, generates the mucus lining in the mouth, throat, lungs, stomach and intestines, and holds the body together. Without the cohesive properties of Kapha, the body would be a pool of disconnected cells scattered on the ground.

Kapha becomes aggravated when the reversed movement of the Vata force reaches the pyloric sphincter - the valve that connects the stomach with the duodenum. Reflux of bile from the gallbladder, as well as toxins and microbes from the intestines, and in some rare cases, even feces, may extend the walls of the duodenum and push through the pyloric sphincter into the stomach. This could lead to various problems associated with digestion.

Stress also aggravates Kapha, which can greatly undermine psychological balance and happiness if disturbed. This is usually accompanied by a 'strange feeling' in the gut and by feelings of insecurity and nervousness.

It is important to remember that every individual has an optimal weight, which is achieved when the body functions at its optimal best. But to rebalance your body's energies and restore your body and mind to their natural state, it is necessary to determine your body type. (Read about this in detail in my book *Timeless Secrets of Health and Rejuvenation*)

Exercise & Body Type

This brings us to the next logical step - body type. Conventionally, there are three body types - ectomorph, mesomorph and endomorph. These body types are based solely on muscle mass and body shape.

The ectomorph is lean and skinny, the mesomorph strong and muscular, and the endomorph round and soft. Thanks to the media, advertising and social conditioning, it is obvious which body type most people long for and try to achieve through dieting and exercise.

Conventional weight-loss programs, with their infamous 'before-and-after' pictures, suggest that with an appropriate diet and set of exercises, every woman can possess a coveted svelte figure and every man can acquire a sculpted muscular physique. It is a great sales pitch aimed where it hurts most - at overweight and obese individuals, many of them desperate to clutch at straws.

But there is a fundamental flaw in this so-called reasoning and classification of body type. It is based solely on external morphological characteristics - shape and size or body mass. Any fitness approach that does not view obesity as a disease but as a physical aberration cannot succeed.

Indeed there are different body types and each one responds differently to food and exercise. But a holistic and natural approach views each one as a sum of the physiological and biochemical processes that constitute each one and the doshas that keep the body alive and breathing.

According to Ayurveda, there are three psycho-physiological body types. Named after the three doshas, they are Vata, Pitta and Kapha.

Vatas generally do well with Yoga, Tai Chi, and Chi Kung. Since Vata types experience energy in bursts, they should be particularly careful not to overexert themselves. When their energy suddenly drops, they can feel depleted for a long time afterward. This often results in depression.

Individuals with a Pitta body type are competitive and are equipped with more drive and energy than Vatas. They prefer a goal-oriented exercise program. However, they also do not have boundless energy and are better off exercising in moderation.

Pittas feel challenged by hiking in the mountains, skiing, jogging, swimming, playing tennis or engaging in other sports that generate in them a sense of achievement.

The unbalanced Pitta type is also a sore loser. Pittas who are easily thwarted should opt for a less competitive exercise program to increase their level of satisfaction. Since excessive heat is a sign of unbalanced Pitta, swimming, which has a cooling influence, is one of the best forms of exercise for them. A walk in the cool forest is another excellent way to pacify an unbalanced Pitta type.

Kapha types are best suited to a good or moderately heavy workout. Weight training, running, rowing, some aerobics, long-distance bicycling, and playing football, basketball and tennis are all suitable for a Kapha.

The Kapha type's steady energy gives him the necessary endurance and stamina to last through long competitive games without feeling tired. Exercise clears out any excessive Kapha congestion, removes excessive water and fat, and improves general circulation.

No two people can exactly be the same because the three bodily doshas are each represented in varied degrees in every person living on the planet. There are, in fact, 10 different body types, most of them a combination of any two doshas.

Having understood that exercise is not about exertion but about energizing the body, it is easy to follow the logic to the next step that along with the correct dietary habits and lifestyle changes, exercise helps rebalance your energies, helps your body self-regulate and restore itself to its optimal weight.

Mind-Body Therapy

I would like to end our discussion on exercise with a brief mention about why yoga is not only an excellent program for good health but for obesity as well. Many people believe that yoga is a slow process that requires supreme patience. That is a popular misconception.

Also the notion that yoga cannot assist in weight loss because it is not strenuous and it doesn't burn fat. This notion stems mainly from the advertising blitz for gyms and aerobics classes which reinforce the belief that you need to perspire profusely to lose weight.

Yoga is one of the most ancient and integrated exercise programs around. It follows the natural principles of the doshas and brings the mind and body in tune with these natural energies.

Apart from the overall health benefits it brings, yoga therapy helps you tune in to the mind-body connection. This is a critical factor for anyone wanting to lose weight because other than the physical aspect, yoga builds a certain mental attitude, which says 'embrace your body'.

An individual who cares for his or her body will stop abusing it through lifestyle, dietary and other choices. This renewed perception of oneself, in mind, body and spirit, is bound to translate into weight loss.

One of the most effective routines in yoga is called the Surya Namaskara or Sun Salutation. This is a series of 12 postures repeated through two cycles. The Surya Namaskara strengthens and stretches all major muscle groups, massages all the internal organs, supports lymph drainage from every part of the body, and enlivens the energy centers and acupuncture points of the body.

This exercise program increases blood flow and circulation, conditions the spine, and improves flexibility of the joints. You may not get the handle on this exercise right from the beginning, but with regular practice you will be able to go through the different positions easily and naturally.

Chapter 13: Burden of Legacy

Grandma used to say: "As you sow, so you shall reap", an adage that perhaps couldn't describe the truth about America's obesity epidemic more appropriately.

Obesity is not a disorder that surfaces overnight. You pave the way for an obese body in childhood. And in the US, the problem has long since reached epidemic proportions.

There is no disputing the fact that we are a nation bringing up generation upon generation of children on fast food, processed food, junk food, high-calorie salted snacks, sweet cookies and candy and sugary beverages that leave the young nutritionally malnourished and overweight.

Perhaps the knee-jerk reaction of most American children to broccoli and other green vegetables being served on the dinner plate is a painful reminder that while our children (those who do sit down for regular meals, that is) gorge on processed beef, chicken, pasta, potato and chili dogs, they are simply not getting sufficient fresh fruit and vegetables.

Add to this the lack of physical activity (using the term 'exercise' might be extreme) among children. The American Heart Association, in fact, lists 'sedentary behavior' among the causes of childhood obesity on its website.

It doesn't take much to guess that too much television viewing, computer usage and video games are the other culprits.

Unhealthy dietary and other habits tend to continue into adulthood, by which time the body has already gone into toxic mode and is responding to a vicious cycle where obesity breeds more obesity.

Also, as if being morbidly obese is not enough, this disease is causing an increasingly large number of children to turn diabetic, a disturbing trend which has emerged only in the last decade.

In fact, according to the Centers for Disease Control (2009), 70 percent of overweight children aged between 5 and

17 have at least one risk factor for heart disease, including elevated blood cholesterol, blood pressure or increased insulin levels. This means, by not taking steps to control your child's weight, you are setting him or her up for hypertension, diabetes, stroke, cancer and osteoarthritis.

The CDC also states that children who are obese are at a greater risk for bone and joint problems, sleep apnea, and social and psychological problems such as stigmatization and poor self-esteem.

The Many Faces of Childhood Obesity

There is no arguing that obesity is a problem of the Western world, a society that is now taking obese children away from their parents and placing them in foster care. Consider these startling cases, which are not often publicly reported due to child privacy laws.

- The latest case (October 2009) is that of a Scottish couple who briefly lost custody for their newborn child after Social Services felt the child was at risk. The couple already had five children, of which two children, aged three and four, had been taken away from them on health grounds. The couple had been told that they might altogether lose custody of their newborn if they failed to bring the weight of their other children under control.
- In May 2009, an American mother from South Carolina lost custody of her 14-year-old son who weighed 555 pounds. The mother was arrested during the custody battle with Social Services, after doctors reported that she had failed to observe measures to rein in his weight. Spooked by the court case, the mother and son fled but were arrested in another state. The teenager is currently living with an aunt and his mother faces criminal child-neglect charges.

- Child custody cases over obesity burst into the public domain in 2007, when a British mother almost lost custody of her morbidly obese eight-year-old son, Connor McCreaddie. The mother eventually worked with local government authorities towards bringing Connor's weight down and was allowed to retain custody of her son. All she did was wean him off processed foods.

Even as more and more custody cases come to light from states such as California, New Mexico, Texas and New York (Canada too has a few), parents, the medico-legal fraternity and child rights advocates are grappling with an issue that is both tricky yet grave.

Some of the questions being asked are: Is morbid obesity is form of child abuse? Should parents lose custody of their obese children on grounds of neglect? The Child Growth Foundation of the UK is lobbying to get the medical community and other experts dealing with children to consider 'overnutrition' as a form of child abuse.

It is a documented fact that childhood obesity can lead to type 2 diabetes (ironically called 'adult-onset' diabetes), insulin resistance, hypertension, sleep apnea, high cholesterol levels, orthopedic problems and the emergence of early puberty due to gross hormonal imbalances.

But while parents are the first to be hauled up, there is perhaps a bigger culprit. Dr Marc S Jacobson, of the Obesity Leadership Work Group of the American Academy of Pediatrics says that childhood obesity isn't always a matter of bad parenting.

He points an accusing finger at the food industry - fast food restaurants, school vending machines, sweetened cereals - all of which are aggressively promoted by food manufacturers and targeted especially at children and adolescents.

Then there are some experts who point out that just as the onus is on parents to raise healthy children, the state too must accept its share of blame. There are some who feel that there is not enough public spending on public parks while others point out that the federal government spends billions of dollars on farm subsidies for poor-quality foods.

But until the government decides to be party to solving America's obesity problem, the onus is on parents to take preventive action. But how can parents do that unless they recognize the problem?

The C S Mott Children's Hospital at the University of Michigan, in a 2007 survey, asked parents to report their oldest child's weight and height and then state whether they thought whether their child was overweight. At a time when child obesity rates are pegged between 13 percent and 17 percent, the results of this survey were astounding.

Around 40 percent of parents of clinically obese children aged between 6 and 11 said their children's weight was "about the right weight". Surprisingly, another 8 percent thought their children were underweight.

A similar survey in Australia found that only 11 percent of parents of overweight five- and six-year-olds, and 37 percent of parents of overweight 10-to-12-year-olds realized that their children had a weight problem.

A British study in 2005 found that less than 2 percent of parents of overweight children aged three to five, and 17 percent of parents of obese children in the same age group recognized that their children had a problem with weight.

Some experts believe that there are so many overweight children in school and elsewhere that perceptions of what is normal weight and what is not have become distorted. Alternatively, some parents go into denial (in a family of overweight people, the yardstick of what is 'normal' tends to change over time).

Today, the US has three times the number of obese children than it did in 1980. But the problem is not distributed evenly. It is linked to economic status, ethnicity and where you live.

According to 2006 statistics of the CDC, 30.7 percent of white American children are overweight or obese, against 34.9

percent of African-American and 38 percent of Mexican American children.

When viewed against income levels, 22.4 percent of 10-to-17-year-olds living below the poverty line (less than $21,200 for a family of four) are overweight or obese, against 9.1 percent of children whose families earn at least four times that much.

When one takes geography into account, 16.5 percent of rural children are clinically obese against 14.4 percent of urban children, according to the 2003 National Survey of Children's Health.

Despite the overwhelming statistics and physical evidence about childhood and adult obesity, the federal and state authorities refuse to step in. But they have made the right moves - on paper at least.

Did you know that there were 400-odd obesity-related bills introduced in state legislatures in the US in 2005? That is more than twice the number in 2003. When it comes to the politics of obesity, it seems our politicians are quicker than ever to appear politically correct.

Consider this. Against the backdrop of this enormous number of obesity-related bills, 25 percent were passed into law in 2005, again double the number from two years before. There have also been suggestions such as putting warning labels on soft drinks and a 'fat tax' on fast food.

But clearly, none of this has made any difference. Americans, children in particular, are gorging on supersized servings of nachos, burritos, pastas, burgers, french fries and colas as much as before while childhood obesity shows no sign of abating.

Dr Robert Lustig, professor of Clinical Pediatrics at UCSF Children's Hospital, says that the Western food environment has become highly 'insulinogenic'. Take a look at the average American's food intake and you will find it full of foods that are high in energy-density, fats, a high glycemic index and fructose, while low in fiber and dairy content. In other words - processed foods and drinks get top billing.

Dr Robert Lustig points out that too much fructose and too little fiber are the cornerstones of America's obesity epidemic due to the way this unhealthy pairing affects insulin. Insulin, a hormone released by the pancreas to assist the absorption of glucose into fuel for the body's cells, acts with another hormone called leptin to control appetite.

Processed foods and junk foods, which took over the American palate 30 years ago, have made the human body insulin and leptin resistant. This is largely due to the addition of sugar and removal of fiber from a wide variety of foods. Foods thus altered are also addictive, Dr Lustig explains.

These food choices are made early on, in childhood. But who is responsible? With their parents usually overweight, overweight and obese children lack healthy role models. With schools dispensing soda, chips and Twinkies through vending machines, is it any wonder that children grow up thinking that these are nutritionally safe choices?

With school lunch rooms serving subsidized processed foods so that the Department of Health can keep food manufacturers happy, can one point an accusing finger at six- and seven-year-olds for growing obese?

It's not that the American Medical Association (AMA) hasn't made the right noises. In 2007, the AMA decided that to make parents 'get the message' that childhood obesity needed to be tackled head-on. It therefore convened a meeting of obesity experts, a meeting that was co-funded by the Department of Health and Human Services and the CDC.

What emerged was a report on childhood obesity that was meant to open the eyes of parents and force them to acknowledge and recognize the seriousness of the problem.

How did it achieve this objective? The AMA, in its wisdom, decided that the language of weight gain had to change. Ten years earlier, children whose Body Mass Index (BMI) was ranked above the 85th percentile for their age were categorized as being 'at risk of overweight'. Doctors were now told not to mince words and simply call these children 'overweight'.

Children with a BMI above the 95th percentile, who were earlier 'overweight', would henceforth be classified as 'obese'. It was a masterstroke at honesty but that is all it was.

Media & TV: Weight and Watch

Most parents and children are probably vaguely aware that too much television watching and computer usage brings on the flab. But most people tend to turn a blind eye to this pressing reality.

Let me present some research findings on the relationship between the television watching (you may include computer usage and video games) and an increase in your child's weight.

- It is an established fact that the number of hours a child spends in front of the television contributes to his or her weight. This has been substantiated by research institutes such as the Johns Hopkins University, the National Cancer Institute and the CDC.

- Researchers at Stanford University have extensively studied body weight differences in third-graders. The study group was told they could watch TV or play video games for a maximum of only seven hours a week. The results showed a significant drop in BMI.

Researchers explain that there are three reasons why TV watching makes children gain weight. One, it reduces physical activity. Two, it leads to an increase in the consumption of sugary drinks and fast food. Three, it lowers the body's resting metabolism or basal metabolic rate.

- As far as the intake of sugary drinks is concerned, one study in 2007 found that with every additional hour of television watched every day, there was an increase in the intake of sugar-sweetened beverages. This amounted to one extra serving per week or a calorie increase of 46.3 per day. If these figures don't seem like a whole lot, they add up over time, not to mention the other harmful changes these toxic beverages produce in the body, and their addictive effects.

While it is correct to assume that physical inactivity means the body burns fewer calories, not many are aware that inactivity - sitting on the couch for hours watching TV - also lowers your resting metabolic rate or basal metabolic rate.

You resting metabolic rate is the rate at which your body uses energy in a post-absorptive state (when not actively digesting food) while at rest. The energy burned in this state is used and needed only to keep your vital organs functioning.

Studies have shown that the body's basal metabolic rate decreases with a decrease in lean body mass and with age. New studies demonstrate that it also decreases with increased television watching.

In effect, this means the more time you spend in front of the television, and if you make this a habit, the fewer calories you burn even when doing nothing!

• Another study of preschoolers found that a child's risk of being overweight increased by 6 percent for every hour of television watched per day. When a television set was present in the child's bedroom, the risk leapfrogged an additional 31 percent for every hour of TV watched.

Researchers also point out that the human body is rapidly developing during childhood, and that the quantum of physical activity is directly correlated with the amount of bone mass the child develops.

• And it is not only the lack of physical activity that is harmful to your child's health. The Kaiser Family Foundation states that very young children cannot distinguish between programming content and advertising. This is a secret weapon used by food and beverage (and many other) manufacturers to brainwash young and vulnerable minds into learning what's healthy and what's not. No prizes for guessing what they're passing off as healthy food choices!

- The US Congress, Children's Television Act of 1990 reports that by the time a child turns 18, he or she has spent between 10,000 and 15,000 hours watching television and has been exposed to more than 200,000 commercials.

- According to the 2004 report 'The Role of Media in Childhood Obesity' by the Kaiser Family Foundation, "during the same period in which childhood obesity has increased so dramatically, there has also been an explosion in media targeted at children: TV shows and videos, specialized cable networks, video games, computer activities and Internet websites." And much of the media targeted to children is laden with elaborate advertising campaigns, many of which promote foods such as candy, soda and snacks.

- The Advertising Coalition states that $10-$15 billion is spent annually on children's food advertising. This roughly translates into 40,000 television commercials a year targeted at children - more than 100 per day. One study recorded 11 food commercials per hour during children's Saturday morning television programming, which means that the average American child is exposed to one food commercial every five minutes! TV commercials directly influence food choices in children. This translates into unhealthy choices - and billions of dollars in profits for food and beverage companies as dietary habits persist into adulthood.

- Did you know that fast food outlets alone spend $3 billion a year on TV commercials specifically aimed at children? And according to 'Advertising, Marketing and the Media: Improving Messages from the Institute of Medicine of the National Academies', food and beverage advertisers together budget for $10-12 billion a year to reach children and the youth.

- Low- and middle-income groups and teenagers from minority communities are most influenced by junk food advertising. Worse still, access to nutritious food is difficult in neighborhoods populated by these communities. Hence, with little access to fruit and vegetable markets, specialty stores and natural food stores, fast food outlets and packaged and processed foods fill a very practical void.

Other Truths about Child Obesity

Mother Knows Best...

Nature intended that every baby be fed on breast milk, and obviously with good reason. Apart from various advantages such as developing healthy immunity in the newborn, breastfeeding may also reduce the risk of childhood obesity.

Researchers at the Harvard School of Public Health say that nursing mothers are more likely to respond to the baby's natural cries and therefore its need for food rather than putting their babies on a schedule. This ensures that the baby is fed proportionate to his or her natural nutritional requirements.

Breast-fed babies also stop eating when they are full while babies brought up on the bottle or formula are fed specific amounts of food and are coaxed to finish what is put in front of them.

...Or Does She?

Specialists in prenatal nutrition believe that pregnant mothers who eat too much junk food could be setting their children up for a life-long battle with the bulge.

A study conducted on rats at the Royal Veterinary College, London, revealed that pregnant rats fed a diet of doughnuts, muffins, chocolate, potato chips, cheese, cookies and candy gave birth to offspring that were fatter, had more muscle waste and showed signs of insulin resistance compared to those who were fed a healthy diet.

Pregnant mothers who gorge on junk food are liable to damage their developing fetuses. Junk foods contain food adulterations and additives and other components such as hydrogenated oils, refined sugars, chemical sweeteners and preservatives.

This increases the chances of the child developing diabetes, heart disease, learning disabilities, cancer and obesity.

Drinking It In Early

Have you ever wondered why some kids remember ad jingles better than they do nursery rhymes or even the alphabet?

Targeting the child consumer is not new but the truth behind child-centered advertising can be scary. And the reason why large corporate firms and advertising agencies are so intent on hooking kids is that the child of today is also tomorrow's consumer.

Child-centered advertising is based on a truth ad agencies (which often hire the expertise of child psychologists) use in a subliminal and devious way: that brand loyalty begins as early as age two.

Going by the diabolical-sounding term, 'cradle-to-grave' advertising, fast food and cola companies realize that children can recognize a brand logo before they can recognize their own name. This explains why marketing logos are designed to be hip and cool and even cartoon-like, so that they impact on young, impressionable and developing minds.

A study published in the Journal of the American Medical Association in 1991 (when Joe Camel ads were all over the media) revealed that almost every American six-year-old could identify Joe Camel, making him as recognizable as Mickey Mouse!

So even if six-year-olds don't smoke at that early age, the assumption cigarette companies make is that they remember 'how cool it is to smoke' later in life. The same reasoning applies to advertisements and logos of soda and cola companies.

Some surveys have found that one-fifth of American one- and two-year-olds drink soda (some are even fed McDonald's milk shake from baby bottles!). Apart from the obvious fat-inducing characteristics of colas, these soft drinks are also addictive due to their caffeine content.

Add a physical craving to brand loyalty at age two and cola companies couldn't ask for more.

But they do. Why else would a popular soft drinks manufacturer license a feeding bottle company to use its logo? As Marion Nestle explains in her book *Food Politics*, the justification used by one soft drinks firm is that using a 'fun logo' would make feeding a fun experience for infants and strengthen the bond between mother and child.

The only truth contained in that sentence is the millions of dollars the soft drinks company had almost ensured it would make with that bit of trickery. After all, studies have shown that parents who use these feeding bottles are more likely to also feed their children soft drinks - just what the cola company had ordered!

'Unconscious' Addiction

We have talked about food cravings (See Chapter 6: Surgery: Fatal Fix) but have you ever wondered what causes food addictions? Why do we salivate at the thought of chicken nuggets and screw up our noses at pumpkin soup?

Perhaps the answer, at least a part of it, lies in 'memes' or tiny bits and pieces of thought, cognition or images that are buried deep in the midbrain. Scientists call memes our 'cultural DNA', which mutate and replicate through the process of cultural selection, comparable to the process of natural selection in the natural world.

When applied to foods and beverages, this is how it works. When a child is introduced to a cola, cookie or a cupcake, and he or she experiences a pleasurable feeling, the brain encodes this as a 'good' or 'positive' stimulus that it would like to experience again.

It does this because the thought or image activates the 'pleasure center' or 'reward center' of the brain which are powered by the neurotransmitter dopamine. This centre of the brain results in feelings of enjoyment and reinforcement and encourages you to repeat the behavior that caused that feeling.

Why did the child experience a pleasurable feeling when he or she first ate the cookie? Either because it was offered as a reward by the parent, was advertised as such or because it tasted similar to other foods he or she had already eaten.

Food and beverage companies in collusion with advertising agencies use subtle but devastating child-centered marketing strategies to trigger a child's pleasure centers even while the child is watching a television commercial. The sole objective, of course, is to 'catch 'em young'.

Processed Poison

We have seen why sugary colas and other soft drinks can be the worst enemy of overweight children. We also know that children are unmindfully raised on colas and other sugary drinks from a tender age.

Researchers have now found a link between overconsumption of sodas and mental health. A study conducted by the University of Oslo, which surveyed 5,000 Norwegian teenagers, found that tenth-graders who drank too much soda were hyperactive and suffered from mental disorders. Also, the more soda the teenager drank, the greater the hyperactivity.

Apart from sodas, parents of children with attention deficit hyperactivity disorder (ADHD), hyperactivity and other behavioral problems should also remove the following from their children's diet: cookies, cupcakes and sugary breakfast cereals.

Processed foods contain vast quantities of chemical additives such as food colorings, which have time and again been linked to ADHD and hyperactivity in children.

In a study commissioned by the Food Safety Agency of the UK, researchers with the University of Southampton further confirmed the association between food colorings and preservatives, and hyperactivity.

Around 300 children were selected for the study and divided into two age groups - one group included children aged three and the other aged eight or nine.

All the children in the sample were fed fruit drinks mixed with either a cocktail of sunset yellow coloring (E110), tartrazine (E102), carmoisine (E122), ponceau 4R (E124) and sodium benzoate (E211) or a mixture of sunset yellow, quinoline yellow (E104), allura red (E129) and sodium benzoate.

The researchers, whose findings were published in the medical journal *The Lancet* in 2008, found that children in both groups exhibited hyperactive behavior. In the younger age group, children who displayed more hyperactivity had consumed the drinks containing the more common combination of chemical agents.

But it isn't just refined sugar and food colorings that do the damage. Refined carbohydrates present in white bread (or food containing refined white flour) such as pasta could aggravate mental disorders like depression, violent behavior and learning disabilities. They also lead to 'brain fog', a condition where the child cannot concentrate on any one thing for very long and feels confused.

Some experts feel consumption of large quantities of refined sugars deprive the body of nutrients critical for neurological health such as the Vitamin B family and minerals including magnesium and zinc.

Alternatively, if your child has a behavioral disorder, it's a good idea to make sure his or her diet includes lots of unprocessed foods like fruit, vegetables, whole grains and super-foods.

As I mentioned earlier, if we take responsibility for our health, if we tune in to our innate wisdom and follow nature's meticulous plan for us, we can heal not only ourselves, but our children as well.

"The natural force within each one of us is the greatest healer of disease." ~ Hippocrates

Author Biography

Andreas Moritz (born January 27, 1954), an American writer born and raised in Southwest Germany, is also a lecturer of Ayurveda, integrative medicine, and mind, body and spirit. He has also specialized in creating fine art as a healing modality. Moritz began his career in Europe as an iridologist (science of eye interpretation) with special focus on identifying and addressing the root causes of illness. He is a former leader of the Transcendental Meditation ('TM') movement. In the mid-1990s, he began publishing self-help books on alternative medicine and mind/body/spirit integration.

Early life, education and accomplishments

From the age of six, Andreas Moritz had to deal with a number of severe illnesses (e.g., juvenile arthritis, arrhythmia, anemia, frequent bouts of passing out [fainting] and irritable bowel syndrome [IBS]). Although his main fields of interest were architecture, music and athletics, he had no choice but to spend the majority of his childhood trying to understand why he was so ill. Accordingly, at age 12, Moritz began studying diet, nutrition and various approaches to natural healing and well-being. In 1970, Moritz began to practice the Transcendental Meditation technique (TM) and Yoga which put an end to his abnormally low blood pressure and regular fainting spells. By age 19, Moritz had fully restored his own health without traditional medicine or outside intervention.

After completing 14 years of primary and higher education in Aalen – a picturesque town in Southwest Germany – Moritz received his 'Abitur' degree at the Schubert Gymnasium, qualifying him to enter university for advanced academic study. In 1974, Moritz completed his seven-month Teacher Training Course, becoming qualified as a teacher of the Transcendental Meditation ('TM') technique. He taught meditation to thousands of people around the world over the course of 20 years.

In 1980, after completing his iridology training by his uncle, Dr. Harry Kirchofer, a leading iridology physician and naturopath in Germany in his time (1914–1996), Moritz proceeded to study and perform research on mind/body medicine at Maharishi European Research University (MERU) in Seelisberg, Switzerland.

In 1981, as part of his training at MERU, Moritz began his studies of **Ayurvedic** medicine. To learn from some of the worlds' most renowned physicians of Ayurveda, including Dr. V.M. Dwivedi, Dr. Balraj Maharishi and Dr. Brihaspati Dev Triguna, Moritz travelled to New Delhi, India (1981–1982). From 1982–1983 Moritz introduced heads of state and members of governments in Ethiopia and Kenya to more holistic and cost effective approaches to healthcare than were available in these impoverished African countries at the time.

In 1991, Moritz finalized his **Ayurveda** training and qualified as a practitioner of Ayurveda (vaidya) in New Zealand.

Moritz lived on the island of Cyprus from 1985–1998, from where he travelled around the world, personally lecturing on and providing alternative healing modalities to governmental leaders who had fallen seriously ill, including the late Prime Minister of Greece, Andreas Papandreou.

Rather than being satisfied with merely treating the symptoms of illness, which typically causes harmful side effects, Moritz dedicated his life's work to understanding and effectively dealing with the root causes of illness, thereby allowing the body to naturally heal itself.

In 1988, Moritz studied and graduated in the Japanese healing art of shiatsu at the British School of Shiatsu in London, England, which has given him insights into the energy systems of the body.

In 1998, Moritz immigrated to Minnesota, in the United States, where he married and began to offer his services to the American people.

As of May 2010, Andreas Moritz is also the author of 12 books, many of which have been translated into several foreign languages, including Russian, Spanish, Chinese, German, Japanese, Greek, Portuguese, French, Dutch and Italian. These include: *Timeless Secrets of Health and Rejuvenation, The Amazing Liver and Gallbladder Flush, Cancer Is Not a Disease! — It's A Survival Mechanism, Lifting the Veil of Duality, It's Time to Come Alive, Heart Disease No More!, Simple Steps to Total Health, Diabetes–No More!, Ending the AIDS Myth, Heal Yourself with Sunlight, Feel Great–Lose Weight,* and *Hear The Whispers–Live Your Dream.*

Moritz has recorded numerous videos and audios on various health and wellness topics, recorded by iHealth-Tube and made available at his web site, www.ener-chi.com. For several years, Andreas ran a free forum 'Ask Andreas Moritz' on the large health website, where over four million readers have read or commented on his messages.

Since taking up residence in the United States in 1999, Andreas has been involved in developing a new and innovative system of healing — called Ener-Chi Art™ — which targets root causes of many chronic illnesses. Ener-Chi Art consists of a series of light ray-encoded oil paintings that can instantly restore vital energy flow (Chi) in the organs and systems of the body. Andreas is also the founder of Sacred Santémony – a powerful system of specially generated frequencies of sound and energy that can transform deep-seated fears, allergies, traumas and mental or emotional blocks into useful opportunities for growth and inspiration within a matter of minutes.

Other Books by the Author

The Amazing Liver and Gallbladder Flush
A Powerful Do-It-Yourself Tool
to Optimize Your Health and Wellbeing

In this revised edition of his bestselling book, *The Amazing Liver Cleanse,* Andreas Moritz addresses the most common but rarely recognized cause of illness - gallstones congesting the liver. Although those who suffer an excruciatingly painful gallbladder attack are clearly aware of the stones congesting this vital organ, few people realize that hundreds if not thousands of gallstones (mainly clumps of hardened bile) have accumulated in their liver, often causing no pain or symptoms for decades.

Most adults living in the industrialized world, and especially those suffering a chronic illness such as heart disease, arthritis, MS, cancer, or diabetes, have gallstones blocking the bile ducts of their liver. Furthermore, 20 million Americans suffer from gallbladder attacks every year. In many cases, treatment consists merely of removing the gallbladder, at the cost of $5 billion a year. This purely symptom-oriented approach, however, does not eliminate the cause of the illness, and in many cases, sets the stage for even more serious conditions.

This book provides a thorough understanding of what causes gallstones in both the liver and gallbladder and explains why these stones can be held responsible for the most common diseases so prevalent in the world today. It provides the reader with the knowledge needed to recognize the stones and gives the necessary, do-it-yourself instructions to remove them painlessly in the comfort of one's own home. The book also shares practical guidelines on how to prevent new gallstones from forming. The widespread success of *The Amazing Liver & Gallbladder Flush* stands as a testimony to the strength and effectiveness of the cleanse itself. This powerful yet simple cleanse has led to extraordinary improvements in health and wellness among thousands of people who have already given themselves the precious gift of a strong, clean, revitalized liver.

Timeless Secrets of
Health and Rejuvenation
Breakthrough Medicine for the 21st Century
(550 pages, 8 ½ x 11 inches)

This book meets the increasing demand for a clear and comprehensive guide that can helps people to become self-sufficient regarding their health and wellbeing. It answers some of the most pressing questions of our time: How does illness arise? Who heals, and who doesn't? Are we destined to be sick? What causes aging? Is it reversible? What are the major causes of disease, and how can we eliminate them? What simple and effective practices can I incorporate into my daily routine that will dramatically improve my health?

Topics include: The placebo effect and the mind/body mystery; the laws of illness and health; the four most common risk factors for disease; digestive disorders and their effects on the rest of the body; the wonders of our biological rhythms and how to restore them if disrupted; how to create a life of balance; why to choose a vegetarian diet; cleansing the liver gallbladder, kidneys and colon; removing allergies; giving up smoking, naturally; using sunlight as medicine; the 'new' causes of heart disease, cancer, diabetes, and AIDS; and a scrutinizing look at antibiotics, blood transfusions, ultrasound scans, and immunization programs.

Timeless Secrets of Health and Rejuvenation sheds light on all major issues of healthcare and reveals that most medical treatments, including surgery, blood transfusions, and pharmaceutical drugs, are avoidable when certain key functions in the body are restored through the natural methods described in the book. The reader also learns about the potential dangers of medical diagnosis and treatment, as well as the reasons vitamin supplements, ;health foods', low-fat products, 'wholesome' breakfast cereals, diet foods, and diet programs may have contributed to the current health crisis rather than helped to resolve it. The book includes a complete program of healthcare, which is primarily based on the ancient medical system of Ayurveda and the vast amount of personal experience Andreas Moritz has gained in the field of health restoration during the past 37 years.

Cancer is Not a Disease!
It's A Survival Mechanism
Discover Cancer's Hidden Purpose, Heal its Root Causes, and be Healthier Than Ever!

In *Cancer is Not a Disease,* Andreas Moritz proves the point that cancer is the physical symptom that reflects our body's final attempt to deal with life-threatening cell congestion and toxins. He claims that removing the underlying conditions that force the body to produce cancerous cells, sets the preconditions for complete healing of our body, mind, and emotions.

This book confronts you with a radically new understanding of cancer - one that revolutionized the current cancer model. On the average, today's conventional 'treatments' of killing, cutting out, or burning cancerous cells offer most patients a remission rate of a mere 7 percent, and the majority of these survivors are 'cured' for just five years or fewer. Prominent cancer researcher and professor at the University of California at Berkeley, Dr. Hardin Jones, stated: "Patients are as well, or better off, untreated..." Any published success figures in cancer survival statistics are offset by equal or better scores among those receiving no treatment at all. More people are killed by cancer treatments than are saved by them.

Cancer is Not a Disease shows you why traditional cancer treatments are often fatal, what actually causes cancer, and how you can remove the obstacles that prevent the body from healing itself. Cancer is not an attempt on your life; on the contrary, this 'dread disease' is the body's final, desperate effort to save your life. Unless we change our perception of what cancer really is, it will continue to threaten the life of nearly one out of every two people. This book opens a door for those who wish to turn feelings of victimhood into empowerment and self-mastery, and disease into health.

Topics of the book include:

- Reasons the body is forced to develop cancer cells
- How to identify and remove the causes of cancer
- Why most cancers disappear by themselves, without medical intervention
- Why radiation, chemotherapy, and surgery never cure cancer
- Why some people survive cancer despite undergoing dangerously radical treatments
- The roles of fear, frustration, low self-worth, and repressed anger in the origination of cancer
- How to turn self-destructive emotions into energies that promote health and vitality
- Spiritual lessons behind cancer

Lifting the Veil of Duality
Your Guide to Living without Judgment

"Do you know that there is a place inside you - hidden beneath the appearance of thoughts, feelings, and emotions - that does not know the difference between good and evil, right and wrong, light and dark? From that place you embrace the opposite values of life as *One*. In this sacred place you are at peace with yourself and at peace with your world." - *Andreas Moritz*

In *Lifting the Veil of Duality,* Andreas Moritz poignantly exposes the illusion of duality. He outlines a simple way to remove every limitation that you have imposed upon yourself during the course of living in the realm of duality. You will be prompted to see yourself and the world through a new lens - the lens of clarity, discernment, and non-judgment. You will also discover that mistakes, accidents, coincidences, negativity, deception, injustice, wars, crime, and terrorism all have a deeper purpose and meaning in the larger scheme of things. So naturally, much of what you will read may conflict with the beliefs you currently hold. Yet you are not asked to change your beliefs or opinions. Instead, you are asked to have *an open mind*, for only an open mind can enjoy freedom from judgment.

Our personal views and worldviews are currently challenged by a crisis of identity. Some are being shattered altogether. The collapse of our current world order forces humanity to deal with the most basic issues of existence. You can no longer avoid taking responsibility for the things that happen to you. When you *do* accept responsibility, you also empower and heal yourself.

Lifting the Veil of Duality shows you how you create or subdue your ability to fulfill your desires. Furthermore, you will find intriguing explanations about the mystery of time, the truth and illusion of reincarnation, the oftentimes misunderstood value of prayer, what makes relationships work, and why so often they don't. Find out why injustice is an illusion that has managed to haunt us throughout the ages. Learn about our original separation from the Source of life and what this means with regard to the current waves of instability and fear so many of us are experiencing.

Discover how to identify the angels living amongst us and why we all have light-bodies. You will have the opportunity to find the ultimate God within you and discover why a God seen as separate from yourself keeps you from being in your Divine Power and happiness. In addition, you can find out how to heal yourself at a moment's notice. Read all about the 'New Medicine' and the destiny of the old medicine, the old economy, the old religion, and the old world.

It's Time to Come Alive!
Start Using the Amazing Healing Powers of Your Body, Mind, and Spirit Today!

In this book, the author brings to light man's deep inner need for spiritual wisdom in life and helps the reader develop a new sense of reality that is based on love, power, and compassion. He describes our relationship with the natural world in detail and discusses how we can harness its tremendous powers for our personal benefit and that of humanity. *It's Time to Come Alive* challenges some of our most commonly held beliefs and offers a way out of the emotional restrictions and physical limitations we have created in our lives.

Topics include: What shapes our destiny; using the power of intention; secrets of defying the aging process; doubting - the cause of failure; opening the heart; material wealth and spiritual wealth; fatigue - the major cause of stress; methods of emotional transformation; techniques of primordial healing; how to increase the health of the five senses; developing spiritual wisdom; the major causes of today's earth changes; entry into the new world; twelve gateways to heaven on earth; and many more.

Simple Steps to Total Health!
Andreas Moritz with co-author John Hornecker

By nature, your physical body is designed to be healthy and vital throughout life. Unhealthy eating habits and lifestyle choices, however, lead to numerous health conditions that prevent you from enjoying life to the fullest. In *Simple Steps to Total Health*, the authors bring to light the most common cause of disease, which is the build-up of toxins and residues from improperly digested foods that inhibit various organs and systems from performing their normal functions. This guidebook for total health provides you with simple but highly effective approaches for internal cleansing, hydration, nutrition, and living habits.

The book's three parts cover the essentials of total health - Good Internal Hygiene, Healthy Nutrition, and Balanced Lifestyle. Learn about the most common disease-causing foods, dietary habits and influences responsible for the occurrence of chronic illnesses, including those affecting the blood vessels, heart, liver, intestinal organs, lungs, kidneys, joints, bones, nervous system, and sense organs.

To be able to live a healthy life, you must align your internal biological rhythms with the larger rhythms of nature. Find out more about this and many other important topics in *Simple Steps to Total Health*. This is a 'must-have' book for anyone who is interested in using a natural, drug-free approach to restore total health.

Heart Disease No More!
Make Peace with Your Heart and Heal Yourself
(Excerpted from Timeless Secrets of
Health and Rejuvenation)

Less than a hundred years ago, heart disease was an extremely rare illness. Today it kills more people in the developed world than all other causes of death combined. Despite the vast quantity of financial resources spent on finding a cure for heart disease, the current medical approaches remain mainly symptom-oriented and do not address the underlying causes.

Even worse, overwhelming evidence shows that the treatment of heart disease or its presumed precursors, such as high blood pressure, hardening of the arteries, and high cholesterol, not only prevents a real cure, but also can easily lead to chronic heart failure. The patient's heart may still beat, but not strongly enough for him to feel vital and alive.

Without removing the underlying causes of heart disease and its precursors, the average person has little, if any, protection against it. Heart attacks can strike whether you have undergone a coronary bypass or have had stents placed inside your arteries. According to research, these procedures fail to prevent heart attacks and do nothing to reduce mortality rates.

Heart Disease No More, excerpted from the author's bestselling book, *Timeless Secrets of Health and Rejuvenation*, puts the responsibility for healing where it belongs, on the heart, mind, and body of each individual. It provides the reader with practical insights about the development and causes of heart disease. Even better, it explains simple steps you can take to prevent and reverse heart disease for good, regardless of a possible genetic predisposition.

Diabetes - No More!
Discover and Heal Its True Causes
*(Excerpted from Timeless Secrets of
Health and Rejuvenation)*

According to this bestselling author, diabetes is not a disease; in the vast majority of cases, it is a complex mechanism of protection or survival that the body chooses to avoid the possibly fatal consequences of an unhealthful diet and lifestyle.

Despite the body's ceaseless self-preservation efforts (which we call diseases), millions of people suffer or die unnecessarily from these consequences. The imbalanced blood sugar level in diabetes is but a symptom of illness, not the illness itself. By developing diabetes, the body is neither doing something wrong, nor is it trying to commit suicide. The current diabetes epidemic is man-made, or rather, factory-made, and, therefore, can be halted and reversed through simple but effective changes in diet and lifestyle. *Diabetes—No More* provides you with essential information on the various causes of diabetes and how anyone can avoid them.

To stop the diabetes epidemic you need to create the right circumstances that allow your body to heal. Just as there is a mechanism to become diabetic, there is also a mechanism to reverse it. Find out how!

This book was excerpted from the bestselling book, *Timeless Secrets of Health and Rejuvenation.*

Ending The AIDS Myth
It's Time to Heal the TRUE Causes!
*(Excerpted from Timeless Secrets of
Health and Rejuvenation)*

Contrary to common belief, no scientific evidence exists to this day to prove that AIDS is a contagious disease. The current AIDS theory falls short in predicting the kind of AIDS disease an infected person may be manifesting, and no accurate system is in place to determine how long it will take for the disease to develop. In addition, the current HIV/AIDS theory contains no reliable information that can help identify those who are at risk for developing AIDS.

On the other hand, published research actually proves that HIV only spreads heterosexually in extremely rare cases and cannot be responsible for an epidemic that involves millions of AIDS victims around the world. Furthermore, it is an established fact that the retrovirus HIV, which is composed of human gene fragments, is incapable of destroying human cells. However, cell destruction is the main characteristic of every AIDS disease.

Even the principal discoverer of HIV, Luc Montagnier, no longer believes that HIV is solely responsible for causing AIDS. In fact, he showed that HIV alone could not cause AIDS. Increasing evidence indicates that AIDS may be a toxicity syndrome or metabolic disorder that is caused by immunity risk factors, including heroin, sex-enhancement drugs, antibiotics, commonly prescribed AIDS drugs, rectal intercourse, starvation, malnutrition, and dehydration

Dozens of prominent scientists working at the forefront of AIDS research now openly question the virus hypothesis of

AIDS. Find out why! *Ending the AIDS Myth* also shows you what really causes the shutdown of the immune system and what you can do to avoid this.

Heal Yourself with Sunlight
Use Its Secret Medicinal Powers to Help Cure Cancer, Heart Disease, Hypertension, Diabetes Arthritis, Infectious Diseases, and much more.

This book by Andreas Moritz provides scientific evidence that sunlight is essential for good health, and that a lack of sun exposure can be held responsible for many of today's diseases.

On the other hand, most people now believe that the sun is the main culprit for causing skin cancer, certain cataracts leading to blindness, and aging. Only those who take the risk of exposing themselves to the sunlight, find that the sun makes them feel and look better, provided they don't use sunscreens or burn their skin. The UV-rays in sunlight actually stimulate the thyroid gland to increase hormone production, which in turn increases the body's basal metabolic rate. This assists both in weight loss and improved muscle development.

It has been known for several decades that those living mostly in the outdoors, at high altitudes, or near the equator, have the lowest incidence of skin cancers. In addition, studies revealed that exposing patients to controlled amounts of sunlight dramatically lowered elevated blood pressure (up to 40 mm Hg drop), decreased cholesterol in the blood stream, lowered abnormally high blood sugars among diabetics, and increased the number of white blood cells which we need to help resist disease. Patients suffering from gout, rheumatoid arthritis, colitis, arteriosclerosis, anemia, cystitis, eczema, acne, psoriasis, herpes, lupus, sciatica, kidney problems, asthma, as well as burns, have all shown to receive great benefit from the healing rays of the sun.

Hear the Whispers, Live Your Dream
A Fanfare of Inspiration

Listening to the whispers of your heart will set you free. The beauty and bliss of your knowingness and love center are what we are here to capture, take in and swim with. You are like a dolphin sailing in a sea of joy. Allow yourself to open to the wondrous fullness of your selfhood, without reservation and without judgment.

Judgment stands in the way, like a boulder trespassing on your journey to the higher reaches of your destiny. Slide these boulders aside and feel the joy of your inner truth sprout forth. Do not allow another's thoughts or directions for you to supersede your inner knowingness, for you relinquish being the full, radiant star that you are.

It is with an open heart, a receptive mind, and a reaching for the stars of wisdom that lie within you, that you reap the bountiful goodness of mother Earth and the universal I AM. For you are a benevolent being of light and there is no course that can truly stop you, except your own thoughts, or allowing another's beliefs to override your own.

May these aphorisms of love, joy and wisdom inspire you to be the wondrous being that you were born to be!

All books are available paperback and as electronic books through the Ener-Chi Wellness Center

Website: http://www.ener-chi.com
Email: support@ener-chi.com
Toll free 1(866) 258–4006 (USA)
Local: 1(709) 570–7401 (Canada)

INDEX

CPSIA information can be obtained at www.ICGtesting.com
Printed in the USA
LVOW090730030712

288673LV00001B/126/P